THE NEUROLOGY OF
DEVELOPMENTAL
DISABILITIES

THE NEUROLOGY OF DEVELOPMENTAL DISABILITIES

By

FRANCIS BENEDICT BUDA, M.D.

Assistant Professor
Neurology and Pediatrics
University Hospital
Jacksonville, Florida

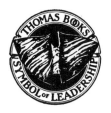

CHARLES C THOMAS • PUBLISHER
Springfield • Illinois • U.S.A.

Published and Distributed Throughout the World by
CHARLES C THOMAS • PUBLISHER
Bannerstone House
301-327 East Lawrence Avenue, Springfield, Illinois, U.S.A.

©*1981, by* CHARLES C THOMAS • PUBLISHER
ISBN 0-398-04373-6
Library of Congress Catalog Card Number: 80-24966

*With THOMAS BOOKS careful attention is given to all details of
manufacturing and design. It is the Publisher's desire to present books that are
satisfactory as to their physical qualities and artistic possibilities and
appropriate for their particular use. THOMAS BOOKS will be true to those
laws of quality that assure a good name and good will.*

Library of Congress Cataloging in Publication Data

Buda, Francis Benedict.
  The neurology of developmental disabilities.

  Bibliography: p.
  Includes index.
  1. Pediatric neurology. 2. Developmental disabili-
ties. I. Title. [DNLM: 1. Child development devi-
ations — Etiology. 2. Child behavior disorders —
Etiology. 3. Nervous system diseases — Infancy and
childhood. 4. Nervous system diseases — Complications.
WS 350.6 B927n]
RJ486.B77   618.92'8   80-24966
ISBN 0-398-04373-6

Printed in the United States of America
C-1

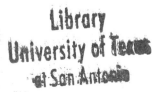

To
my daughter
Catherine SaraAnne

PREFACE

THIS BOOK is designed to honestly discuss the varied manifestations of pathological conditions that may affect the immature nervous system and produce a developmental disability. All individuals with developmental disabilities have some dysfunction of their central nervous system. In some instances, gross pathological changes can be identified, but, more often, no anatomical defect can be seen on pathological study of the brain. Yet, some pathological process must exist on a neuronal level or as a defect with intercellular connection. In the developmentally disabled, the defective nervous system acts as an unexposed, enclosed controlled system that produces overt problems in other areas of the body. Too often, professionals focus on the overt secondary symptom without the full appreciation of the primary defect that is within the nervous system.

Through my work as a pediatric neurologist on developmental evaluation teams, as a consultant to a large state hospital for the developmentally disabled, and as chief of professional education at that same facility, my experience with the many professionals who work with the developmentally disabled has broadened. From this experience, my attention has been focused on the paucity of understanding by many professionals for the neurological basis of developmental disabilities. The purpose of this book is to aid these professionals in their understanding.

Organizationally, the book is divided into chapters dealing with specific clinical symptoms or groups of diseases. The reader should be cautioned that an individual may have only one problem or may have several problems, e.g. seizure disorder, right hemiparesis, and hyperactivity. If several problems exist, they are almost always manifestations of a single event or process that lead to the dysfunction of the central nervous system producing several clinical manifestations. This individual may be at risk for other disabilities as maturation of the nervous system progresses and developmental milestones are anticipated, e.g. acquisition of reading skills. Although little can be done to prevent the disability from becoming manifested, early diagnosis and intervention may help to minimize the severity of the deficit.

This book is written for all professionals who work with the developmentally disabled. It is my hope that knowledge of neuro-developmental pathophysiology will lead to a better understanding of the varied conditions called developmental disabilities. It is with this understanding that realistic treatment planning can be made, and realistic expectations can be achieved.

ACKNOWLEDGMENTS

Mentors: Doctor Edward Rabe, Tufts-New England Medical Center Hospitals, whose developmental and clinical approach to diagnosis served as a personal guide for patient management and inspiration for this book. Doctor Thomas Twitchell, Tufts-New England Medical Center Hospitals, from whom the author gained insight into development and cerebral palsy. Doctor Floyd Gilles, Harvard-Boston Children's Hospital, whose emphasis on primary understanding of pathology and critical analysis of established thinking has served the author as a model for the assessment of the conditions discussed in this book.

Fellow Professionals: Many diverse individuals from different professions have devoted much of their lives to the care of the developmentally disabled. The author's admiration for the self-less work of individuals such as Mrs. Donna Jackson, Ms. Sima Siskind and Doctor Richard Skinner has served as a motivation for the preparation of this book.

Patients: Many patients have contributed to the author's understanding of the nature of developmental disabilities and provided an impetus for the conception of this book, with special appreciation to Brian, Tracie, Joshua, and Catherine.

Personnel at University Hospital of Jacksonville: Doctor Ronald Rhatigan, Doctor Louis Russo and Ms. Mel Lewis have contributed their support for the preparation of this book. Much appreciation for the assistance of the Medical Photography Department with grateful acknowledgment to Mrs. Gladys Donaroma for her preparation of illustrations and Mark A. Hildreth for his photographic work. The invaluable secretarial assistance and interest of Ms. K. Miriam Sorensen is very deeply appreciated.

F. B. B.

CONTENTS

xi

LIST OF ILLUSTRATIONS

LIST OF TABLES

THE NEUROLOGY OF
DEVELOPMENTAL
DISABILITIES

Chapter 1

A DEVELOPMENTAL APPROACH TO DEVELOPMENTAL DISABILITIES

T HE DEFICIT produced when a developing nervous system is injured is different than when a mature nervous system is damaged. When the mature nervous system is damaged the deficit becomes readily apparent. When an immature nervous system is damaged, the areas that are damaged may not be serving a demonstrable function at the time of the insult, but would do so only as the individual matures. In severe injury, function may never develop. However, in most instances, the area is not completely destroyed and what results is a lag in the development of the functional area that has been damaged. Therefore, the involved function does develop, but it develops at a slower rate than normal and usually attains a less sophisticated final level of performance. This type of injury to an immature nervous system produces what is termed a *developmental lag*.[1]

The concept of developmental lag applies to any developing functional area in an immature nervous system that is damaged regardless of the etiology of the damage. For example, a child who has suffered damage in the area of gross motor performance may not be able to achieve his major gross motor landmarks at the normal age. Although he may not be able to walk by twelve to eighteen months of age[2] he may be able to walk (example in Figure 1) by thirty-six months of age. This represents a developmental lag in the area of gross motor performance.

Most individuals who have experienced damage to their developing nervous system are not in a static state, but are in a state of change where the rate is slower than normal. What the damaged infant or child and the normal have in common is they both have a constantly changing baseline of motor and intellectual performance. The retarded infant by definition progresses at a slower rate and often plateaus at an earlier age than normal.

3

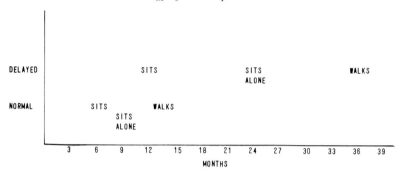

Figure 1. Timetable for normal gross motor development and an example of delayed gross motor development.

These children with retarded development do not as a rule *catch up* to their normal peers, but both the normal child and the child with retardation share a changing baseline of motor and intellectual performance.

Understanding the concepts of developmental lag and changing baseline are of paramount importance to the understanding of many of the difficulties seen in the developmentally disabled. In Figure 1 we see the normal timetable for gross motor development with the infant sitting when placed at six months of age, sitting alone at nine months of age and walking around at twelve to eighteen months of age.[2, 3] He has a changing baseline of gross motor performance. Also, in Figure 1, we have an example of a child with a developmental lag in the acquisition of gross motor skills. His timetable indicates that he will sit when placed at twelve months of age, sit alone at twenty-four months of age, and walk alone at thirty-six months of age. He too has a changing baseline of gross motor performance, but he has a developmental lag in the acquisition of gross motor skills.

These concepts of developmental lag and changing baseline make one look with skepticism upon methods of reflex patterning that allege to facilitate development. They would infer that introduction of therapy in our example (Figure 1) at nine months of age in a child who is not sitting will produce the gross motor landmarks of sitting, sitting alone, and finally walking alone at thirty-six months, but do not consider the individual's innate changing baselines of performance. Regardless of whether the child received therapy, his innate timetable would dictate walking to occur at thirty-six months. No controlled study has ever shown that methods of intervention of reflex patterning that allege to facilitate development have been successful.[4] It has been shown that adequate stimulation is as important as formalized therapy to allow the individual to rapidly achieve his full potential.[5]

Many of the problems seen in the developmentally disabled can be viewed in a developmental framework. A knowledge of the normal developmental sequence of certain functions can be exceedingly useful in putting many of these problems into their proper perspective. In actuality, the study of the retarded infant or child has contributed significantly to our understanding of the normal physiological development, particularly with reference to the motor system.

Gross Motor Development

The normal timetable for gross motor development is shown in Table I. This starts off in the infantile period with the infant

Table I

TIMETABLE OF NORMAL GROSS MOTOR DEVELOPMENT AND PREDICTIVE AUTOMATISMS

Task	*Age*
A. Gross body postural development	
Infantile posture	0-4 weeks
Asymmetric tonic neck posture	4 weeks to 4 months
Sitting when placed	6 months
Sitting alone	9 months
Cruising	9-11 months
Walking alone	12-18 months
B. Development of leg and foot automatisms	
Neonatal placing	0-4 months
True anterior placing	4 months
Medial and lateral placing	6 months
Posterior placing	9 months
C. Hand motor development	
Infantile posture	0-4 weeks
Holding of object when placed in hand	2 months
Midline grasping	4 months
Full fisted reach and grasp	6 months
Pincer grasp	9-11 months
D. Development of hand automatisms	
Contact grasp	2 months
Instinctive grasp orientation phase	6 months
Full development of instinctive grasping	9 months

lying in a very characteristic posture (Figure 2).[2] While supine, the infant prefers to lie with his arms flexed and his ankles dorsiflexed. The infant is not frozen in this position but prefers to lie in this position for the first four weeks of life. At four weeks of age this posture gives way to the asymmetric tonic neck posture (Figure 3), which is the predominant body posture from four weeks to four months of age.[2, 3] In this posture, when the infant lies supine and turns his head to one side, the side to which the occiput is pointing will flex (both arm and leg), and the side to which the nasion is pointing will extend (both arm and leg). The infant is not frozen in this posture, but will tend to lie in this posture at rest. Finally, the asymmetric tonic neck posture gives way to the sitting posture at six months in which the child will sit when placed. The child will sit alone at nine months, will walk

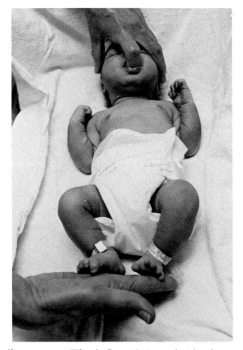

Figure 2. Infantile posture. The infant (0-4 weeks) in the supine position lies with elbows, wrists, and fingers flexed, his knees flexed and his ankles dorsiflexed.

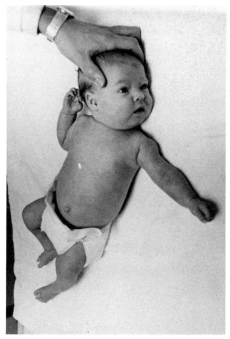

Figure 3. The asymmetric tonic neck posture. When the head is turned to the side, the side to which the occiput is pointing will flex (both arm and leg) and the side to which the nasion points will extend (both arm and leg).

holding on at nine to eleven months and will finally walk alone by twelve to eighteen months.[2]

Often it is useful to be able to predict whether or not a child is ready to walk. There are certain automatisms, developmental reflexes which occur at prescribed time periods, that lead in a sequential fashion to the acquisition of the walking skill. If the neonate were to be suspended in midair (Figure 4a) and the anterior aspect of his foot touched to a surface, he will pick his legs up in the air (Figure 4b) and place them down flat on the surface (Figure 4c). This automatism is present for the first two months of life. At four months of age, this gives way to a *true anterior placing response* where, if the infant is suspended and the anterior aspect of his foot touched to a surface (Figure 5a), he will orient his foot to the shape of the surface until he reaches the

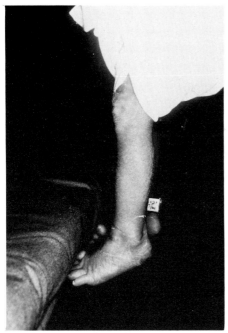

Figure 4A

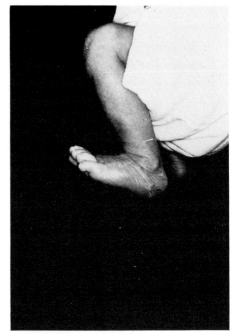

Figure 4B

Figure 4. The infantile placing response. In 4A the infant is suspended and the anterior aspect of his foot is placed in contact with a surface. In 4B he reflexly picks up his legs and in 4C he places them flatly upon the surface.

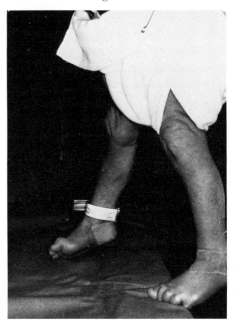

Figure 4C

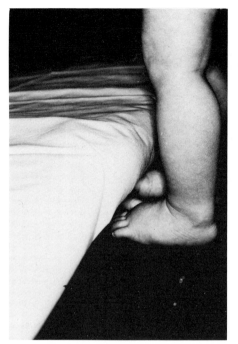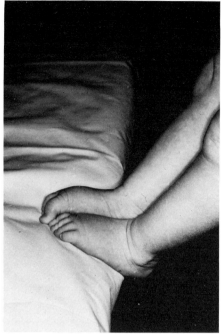

Figure 5. The true anterior placing response. In 5A the infant is suspended and the anterior aspect of his foot is placed in contact with a surface, and, in 5B, he orients his foot to the shape of the surface.

top (Figure 5b). This differs from the neonate who has no regard to the contour of the surface. At six months of age, if one were to stimulate the medial or lateral aspect of the child's foot to a surface he would do the same orientation maneuver to reach the top. Finally, at nine months of age, if one were to touch the posterior aspect of his foot to a surface, he would orient his foot to it until he reaches the top. The acquisition of the posterior placing automatism precedes the child's ability to walk and can be used as an indicator of when a child is ready to acquire the gross motor act of walking.[7]

There is also a normal developmental pattern of hand function that follows an orderly developmental sequence in the normal child and in the child with a delay in gross hand motor development. Again, at birth, the child prefers to lie with his

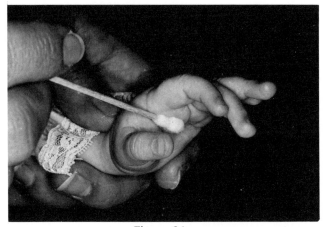

Figure 6A

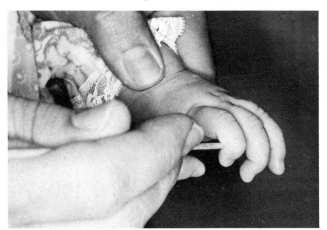

Figure 6B

Figure 6. The contact grasp. In 6A the stimulus is introduced to the proximal portion of the hand and as it moves distally the infant grasps it as in 6B.

wrist flexed and his fingers flexed in the infantile posture (Figure 2).[2] However, at two months of age, this posture is relaxed and an object can be placed in his hand and he will hold onto it and use it for self-stimulation.[3] At four months of age, the infant is capable of making grasping motions toward the midline and will achieve some midline grasping.[3] This is in contrast to the six month old who is able to reach out with a full fist laterally and grasp an object.[3] By nine to eleven months of age, the grasp becomes sufficiently sophisticated to achieve a pincer grasp where the thumb and index finger can be opposed.[3]

There are some definite predictors of when an individual will be able to achieve some of his developmental landmarks. At two months of age, when the child's hand is held in a very neutral position and a distally moving stimulus is introduced (Figure 6a); as the stimulus moves distally the child will flex his fingers and grasp onto the object (Figure 6b). This is called the contact grasp and is acquired at two months of age and precedes the child's ability to hold onto an object when it is placed in his hand.[8] Therefore, in a child with a developmental lag, if one is questioning when it would be appropriate to introduce stimuli to be held in the hand for self-stimulation, one would test for the contact response.

At five to six months of age the first phase of instinctive grasping arises.[8] To test for this, a stimulus is introduced either to the medial or lateral aspect of the child's hand, and the child will orient his hand to the side of the stimulus (Figure 7a). This is accomplished totally independent of sight. The acquisition of this first phase of instinctive grasping precedes the child's ability to reach out laterally with a full-fisted grasp for objects. To determine when it would be fruitful to introduce objects into a child's field for the stimulation of the full-fisted lateral grasping response, one would check for the first phase of instinctive grasping.

Instinctive grasping goes through other stages until it becomes fully developed by nine months of age, at which point not only will the child orient his hand to a stimulus which is introduced on the medial or lateral aspect of the hand but will grope (Figure 7b) and finally grasp the stimulus totally independent of sight (Figure 7c). It is the full development of the instinctive grasp response that precedes the child's ability to reach out with the thumb and index finger (pincer grasp) for fine objects.[7] Testing for a fully developed instinctive grasp response is useful in determining whether or not a child is ready to start reaching out for pellets, e.g. raisins, cereal.

Through the use of these automatisms, we have the ability to

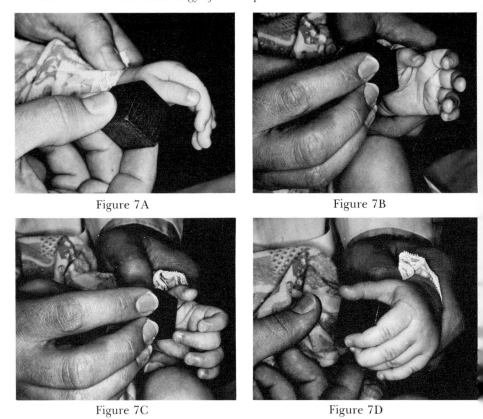

Figure 7A   Figure 7B

Figure 7C   Figure 7D

Figure 7. The instinctive grasp. A stimulus is introduced to the medial aspect of an infant's hand in 7A. He then orients his hand to the stimulus in 7B, gropes after the stimulus in 7C and grasps it in 7D, all independent of sight.

stage the gross motor development of the child, either normal or delayed, and predict when some of the major landmarks will be achieved.

Neuromuscular Coordination

Just as there is a normal timetable for gross motor development, there is a normal timetable for the acquisition of fine coordinative skills. Children who have a delay in their neuromuscular coordination often come to the physician's attention by the time they enter kindergarten; at this point in their life, their teacher is requiring the child to perform some acts that require fine coordination such as coloring within lines, manipulating scissors, or tying shoe laces. The parents may become aware of difficulty at this stage because the child may not perform the fine coordinative tasks that his peers are capable of doing.

Although an individual may have difficulty with fine coordinative tasks, it is often difficult to accurately evaluate this on testing. In Table II, there is a series of simple tasks that can be tested to determine if a child's fine coordinative skills are appropriate for his age level.[9, 10] Also, in Table II, historical factors are included, riding a tricycle at three years of age and riding a bicycle without training wheels at six years of age.

Unfortunately, if someone has a lag in his neuromuscular coordinative development, little can be done to facilitate their progress except for building confidence, since there is an innate changing baseline for the development of fine coordinative skills.[17] Inferring that special programs facilitate fine coordinative development lacks physiological proof. Children who have delay in neuromuscular coordination are not in a static state, but are developing according to their own changing baseline of fine coordinative performance.[12]

Table II
TIMETABLE OF FINE NEUROMUSCULAR COORDINATION

Age in Years	Task
1.5	Smooth eye tracking.
3	Labial, lingual and gutteral sounds.
	Rides tricycle.
5	Head-eye dissociative movements.
	Serial apposition of fingers.
	Rapid alternating hand movements with outstretched arms.
	Rapid heel to shin movements.
	Hopping on either foot.
5-6	Rides bicycle without training wheels.
7	Performs serial rapid fire commands.
	Right-left orientation.
	Alternate cheek puffing.
8	Raises eyebrows.
	Performs fine rapid tongue movements.

Table III

TIMETABLE OF NORMAL SPEECH DEVELOPMENT

Age in Months	Task
2-4	Babbling
6-9	Repetitive syllables
9-12	Repetitive syllables with meaning
12-18	Whole words
24	Phrases

Speech

There is a normal timetable for the acquisition of speech skills.[2, 3] The etiology of delayed speech is variable. Etiologies include deafness, articulation defects, psychosocial factors, etc.[13, 14] In the developmentally disabled, the delay in speech is often based on a lag in the development of the speech areas of the brain. In this instance, the child's speech would follow the pattern of normal development of speech (Table III), but it would achieve the developmental stages at a much slower pace. It is very important to define the rate of progress a child is making in his speech when one assesses a child with a speech difficulty, since instituting an elaborate speech therapy program would be inappropriate for a child with a simple developmental lag in the acquisition of speech skills. Such programs may actually lead to greater frustration for the child and for his family.

Reading

Reading is a complicated act that can be broken down into many different operations including the discrimination of forms, the discrimination of form orientation in space, the discrimination of form sequence, the remembering of each of these factors, and the ability to focus attention on a whole word.[15] A child who manifests a difficulty in reading may have a deficit in any of these areas and have a reading difficulty.

Often reading difficulties result from a developmental delay in the acquisition of reading skills. One of the clues to this type of difficulty in a child is the reversal of letters or the reading of mirror word forms, e.g. reading *was* as *saw*. When three-to-five-year-old children were taught reading and writing, it was found that they reversed letters and words.[17] There is no difficulty when one reverses or mirrors an *e* or an *s* but there is difficulty when one mirrors or reverses a *p* or a *b* because the mirror symbol has a different meaning. Apparently, the child who reverses does not really discriminate a difference between letters written in their mirror image. If a child manifests this difficulty past the age of seven it usually indicates a developmental lag in acquiring the reading skills.[1] This does not mean that the child would be incapable of reading in the future. It usually indicates that he is delayed in acquiring reading skills but should acquire some level of reading as he matures. Again, intensive programming for the child with this type of difficulty may lead to frustration, but a program of reading readiness that would address the child at the level he is functioning would yield better results.

However, the children who have difficulty in the discrimination of forms, serial ordering of forms, orientation of forms in space, or in focusing attention on each word require special types of intervention. Therefore, when dealing with the child who has difficulty in reading it would be important to determine which pattern of difficulty he manifests because that would determine the type of remediation he should receive.

All children with reading difficulties are often termed *dyslexic*. The term *dyslexia* only means trouble reading and is not a diagnostically definitive term. All children with dyslexia are not alike and should not be treated in the same manner (see Chapter 11).

Hyperactivity

Hyperactivity is a symptom, not a diagnostic entity. This symptom can be viewed in a framework of being either primary or secondary to other factors neurologic and psychogenic.[18] Many individuals who manifest the problem of *primary* (also called developmental) hyperactivity really are thought to show a developmental lag in the acquisition of control of their activity level.[19] To support this hypothesis of primary hyperactivity one would look at the normal progression of activity in children. The toddler (terrible two's) is very restless and distractable. The preschool age child is less active and less distractable. The school age child is less active than the preschooler. Therefore it is possible to look at primary hyperactivity as a developmental lag in acquiring the skill of activity level control (see Chapter 10).

Many of the problems seen in the developmentally disabled can be viewed in a developmental perspective. Each individual whether he is normal or delayed has an internal timetable for a changing baseline of motor and intellectual performance. The normal child has one timetable and the delayed child has another. In general, neither is in a static state. Children with retardation in areas of motor or intellectual performance will be delayed in acquiring those developmental landmarks. Although individuals may be delayed in one area, they may not necessarily be delayed in others, although they are at risk for having delays in acquiring other skills. The delays seen in the child with developmental disability reflects some damage to the central nervous system which occurred before the involved performance area functionally began to mature.

Chapter 2

SPECIAL TECHNIQUES IN THE NEUROLOGICAL EXAMINATION OF THE DEVELOPMENTALLY DISABLED

THE TWO MOST IMPORTANT tools in the neurological examination of a child with developmental disabilities are a keen sense of observation and a knowledge of what the normal performance standards are for children at given chronological ages so that tests appropriate for their age can be used to obtain information. It is important to address the child at his developmental age rather than his chronological age for testing. For this reason, a quick assessment of the child's developmental level is useful information to obtain at the outset of the evaluation. A simple developmental sequence is provided (*see* Table IV) which will enable one to stage a child's development within a few minutes.[2, 3, 9, 10, 21]

Many individuals performing neurological assessments on patients with developmental disabilities will search carefully for soft neurological signs. Soft neurological signs are those that can only be elicited by special maneuvers and/or are developmentally normal for a given age, but would have disappeared at the patient's current chronological age.[1] An example of a soft neurological sign would be a child who postures his arms in the infantile posture (Figure 2) upon prolonged heel or toe walking. This is a normal phenomenon until the age of five, but after five years of age, posturing of both arms would be a soft neurological sign of generalized immaturity, and posturing of just one arm would be a sign of neurological dysfunction of one side of the body.

For ease in understanding, this chapter is divided into sections including: appearance, developmental evaluation, cranial nerves, motor functions, sensory examination, cerebellar functions (coordination), gait and station, and head.[22] Testing for

17

each of these areas is discussed according to chronological age where applicable.

Appearance

So very much information can be obtained by simply critically observing the activity of a child. Not only can one gain insight into how he interacts with his surroundings and other people, but also one can begin to get some insight into how his nervous system is functioning. For example, if one sees that the child is lying quietly in the bed but only using the left side of his body and not using the right side of his body it would make one suspicious that there is some dysfunction on the right side. If someone is immersing himself in a task that is more appropriate for someone of a lower chronological age it would make one suspicious that the child's intellectual level is depressed. During the period of observation, one is looking at what the child is doing and how he is moving various parts of his body. Is he moving in a smooth coordinated fashion? Are his movements jerky or tremulous? Is he having involuntary movements along with regular motions? Does he have any particular posturing of one part of his body?

One should observe the child's state of consciousness. Is this child in contact with his environment? Does he have brief lapses or periods when he seems to stare blankly into space? Is he having brief seizures? Children who are having absence spells (petit mal) may have brief periods of staring into space which interrupt the normal activity they are undertaking, but they will resume the activity after the brief period of staring has abated.[23] Is the child carrying on one repetitive act? Does he relate to other individuals or children in his environment? A child who has autistic behavior would not relate to other children or adults in a way that is any different than he would relate to a chair or a table in a room.

This period of quiet observation may lead to the child becoming aware of the examiner's presence. The examiner may be able to make an introduction into the child's play world. In this way he may begin to gain the child's confidence and start his examination. If the child is uncooperative, the information that one can obtain from the examination becomes somewhat limited. The first step in doing an accurate neurological examination is to put the child at ease and to begin to interact with the child in a nonthreatening way.

From the observation period one should note the child's general physical characteristics. Are there any dysmorphic features in the child? Are his growth parameters, height and weight, appropriate for his age? What are the relative sizes of his limbs? Are they symmetrical? Is one side of the body underdeveloped compared to the other? Are his legs underdeveloped compared to his torso and arms? Are there any congenital anomalies that are apparent of his extremities or body? Does he have enlarged organs, e.g. liver or spleen? Does he have any body deformities? Particular attention should be paid to the child's skin. Does he have any areas of increased pigmentation or areas of decreased pigmentation or peculiar rashes or peculiar coloration to his skin? All of these may give one clues to certain diseases that are associated with developmental disabilities. For example, the occurrence of hypopigmented and raised rough chagrin patches are seen in tuberosclerosis (see Appendix C).

During the observation period, the critical observer begins to formulate a general impression of the child's social and developmental skills. At the same time, he is gathering information about the child's morphology, looking for diagnostic clues and putting the child at ease before proceeding to the more formal portions of the examination.

A general principle when examining infants and children is to start with the least uncomfortable procedure and progress to the more uncomfortable ones.

Developmental Examination

No neurological examination of a developmentally disabled individual would be complete without a brief assessment of development. If detailed testing is needed, the child should be referred to a psychologist for evaluation. However, there is a very simple schema that one can use (Table IV) with which one can quickly stage the infant's or child's development.[2, 3, 9, 10] With the exception of speech and reading,[21] none of the testing used in this schema relies on prior learning. In this way, therefore, the cultural and environmental biases to testing are minimized.

Cranial Nerves

Olfactory

This is the first cranial nerve. It is difficult to test unless there is patient cooperation since this nerve controls our sense of smell. In order to test it, a stimulus such as peppermint or dry coffee is introduced to the patient with his eyes closed. The patient is then asked what he smells. This is done with one nostril occluded and the test repeated with another stimulus as the other nostril is occluded. In individuals who cannot cooperate, examiners attempt to test this cranial nerve with a noxious odor to see if the patient responds. When this is done, one is really testing the sensory part of cranial nerve V which discriminates painful stimuli from the skin and mucus membranes of the head.

Optic

The second cranial nerve is the optic nerve. It is this nerve that enables us to appreciate visual stimuli. From the time of birth, full-term infants are capable of fixing and following objects. The newborn follows in a very characteristic manner. He is capable of following a stimulus from the midline laterally or medially and back to the midline. Crossing the midline with the stimulus is exceedingly difficult for the newborn infant. This is a skill he acquires at approximately one to two months of age and certainly by three months of age.[3]

Much information can be gained by looking into the fundus (the back part of the retina). In doing this, one needs to use an ophthalmoscope and look through the pupil to appreciate whether or not there are any opacities in the cornea or the lens. In looking at the optic nerve head one gets a chance to actually look at a part of the central nervous system. Also, one gets a chance to look at the blood vessels in this area and check if there are any hemorrhages or any abnormal configurations of blood vessels. In addition, one is looking for areas of accumulated white material or for areas of increased pigmentation.[24]

Occasionally, it is important to check for a child's ability to see objects in his lateral visual fields. In children over five years this can be accomplished as in an adult by checking for latent finger motion while the person fixes on an object in the center of his visual field.[24] In infants and younger children this can be accomplished by diverting the child's attention to an object in the center of his visual field and then introduce objects from behind his head and bring them forward until the child responds to their presence.[22]

Oculomotor, Trochlear, and Abducens

The third, fourth, and sixth cranial nerves control the muscles required for eye movement. The third cranial nerve also controls the pupillary size and its response to light and accommodation. One would look to see if the pupils are equal, note their configuration and how they react to light. Individuals may have some pupillary unrest, which means that when one shines the light in their pupil, instead of the pupil constricting, the pupil will alternately constrict and dilate. When individuals are having seizures, it is common to see severe pupillary unrest.[25]

The extraocular muscles control the way our eyes can move in all planes of vision. Some information concerning the muscles can be obtained by having the individual fix and follow on an object.[25] For a newborn baby, large objects like one's face or a 5 cm red disc may be used to check the extraocular muscles. If the infant is uncooperative, one may perform an oculocephalic maneuver (turning the infant's head from side to side) while holding the eyes open. The reflex response is for the infant's eyes to move in the direction opposite the movement of the head. This can be accomplished in the horizontal and vertical planes.

Another way to test this is by picking up the infant and gently spinning him in an arc. This maneuver will usually reflexly cause the infant to open his eyes and produce the same eye movement as the oculocephalic response. Either of these maneuvers will also check for the integrity of the vestibular portion of the eighth cranial nerve.[2]

Later in infancy any brightly colored object will suffice for checking extraocular muscles. Very often a finger puppet can be quite useful in getting a young child to fix on an object and follow. Usually by the time a child is developmentally five years of age, he is capable of performing voluntary finger following as one would use in testing an adult for the mobility of the extraocular muscles.

Trigeminal

The fifth cranial nerve has both sensory and motor components. The motor component will control our muscles of mastication. These muscles are responsible for chewing and in infants for sucking. They can be checked for in a newborn without teeth by inserting one's finger in the baby's mouth and seeing how well he is capable of sucking or masticating on the finger. Later on in life one can check the child's ability to chew and at the same time feel how well he moves the muscles which control his jaw. In addition, a concrete way of checking motor cranial nerve V is to check for the jaw jerk. The jaw jerk is checked like a deep tendon reflex by gently percussing the chin with the mouth slightly opened and watching for a reflex closure of the mouth.

The sensory portions of the fifth cranial nerve control all of our sensations of touch and pain about the face. There are three divisions of this: the ophthalmic, which supplies the area above the lateral aspect of the canthus (where the upper and lower eyelid meet latently); the maxillary, which controls the area between the lateral border of the canthus to the upper border of the mouth; and the mandibular, which controls the area of the lower part of the face below the lower lip.[26] In order to check for these sensory components of the fifth cranial nerve, one can, in a person who is cooperative, have him close his eyes and gently stroke those areas of the face with a piece of cotton. The person is asked to state when he feels the stimulus. For pain testing, one can use a pin and find if the patient is capable of perceiving pain. However, this is quite difficult in someone under approximately five years of age. The corneal reflex is one that is initiated by sensory stimulus to the cornea (which is supplied by the fifth cranial nerve) causing the person to blink. The stimulus is usually a sterile piece of cotton with which one can confidently test ophthalmic division of sensory V. The rooting response, which is present from birth until four months of age in the awake state and from birth to seven months of age in the drowsy state,[3] can be used to test for touch sensation. This is a response that relies upon light touch for its initiation, and one can stimulate it in the superior quadrant of the mouth or the inferior quadrant of the mouth. If the rooting response is initiated, one can be confident that touch can be perceived in the maxillary and mandibular division of sensory cranial nerve V.

Facial

The seventh cranial nerve supplies the muscles that enable us to move the different portions of our face. Much information concerning the function of the seventh cranial nerve can be gained by keen observation. Does the person wrinkle both sides of his forehead symmetrically? Does he close both eyes with equal intensity? When he smiles do his lips move symmetrically? At rest, is one palpebral fissure larger? Asymmetries often indicate some dysfunction on one side. Good keen observation is really very important, particularly in someone who is functioning in the newborn period of life where cooperation for making facial movements on command is limited. Even later in the infantile period cooperation is rather poor for a child to move his face about on command. Only when the child reaches between three and five years of age can he carry out facial movements on command. In the newborn period, more information can be obtained by using the rooting response. If one were to stimulate the rooting response, one could observe whether or not the child will move his cheek towards the side of the stimulus. This would be a good check to see if there is good muscle strength in the lower facial muscles.

Acoustic

The eighth cranial nerve supplies our sense of hearing as well as our sense of balance.[26] In order to check for hearing one really needs the cooperation of the person. There are some detailed tests done by the otologist where the person can be placed in a room and checked to see if he activates to sounds introduced into one or the other ear. In the newborn, this is an exceptionally difficult phenomenon to check when one is looking for activation of the child following a sound. One must be cautious that visual stimuli or air current movement are not introduced since they may produce a response of head turning. In a cooperative person, one may even be able to do the Rinne[27] and Weber tests[28] which enable one to determine whether or not there is normal acoustic nerve function and normal air conduction. The Rinne test, which presents a sound by air and then bone conduction, determines whether air conduction or bone conduction is better. The Weber test places the stimulus (a tuning fork) in the center of the forehead to determine if it is lateralized to one side or the other. The nerve functions better on the side on lateralization except in conductive hearing losses where the sound is appreciated better on the side of the conductive defect. In checking for the vestibular component of the eighth cranial nerve, one would do an oculocephalic or a doll's eye maneuver. In the newborn period, one would rotate the child's head, maintaining the eyes open (see Oculomotor, Trochlear, and Abducens above).

Glossopharyngeal and Vagal

There is a limited amount of simple testing for these cranial nerves considering the extent of their innervation, but most of their innervation is in areas that are not readily accessible to examination.[26] One can depress the patient's tongue with a tongue blade and look to see if the uvula is midline. The person should then be stimulated in the posterior pharynx with the tongue blade on the left and then on the right. This is done to determine if the person perceived the stimulus and will gag and whether he is capable of elevating the uvula in the midline.

Spinal Accessory

The eleventh cranial nerve controls the muscles of the upper part of the neck and some of the back.[26] The muscle that is often checked for is the sternocleidomastoid, which controls the head movement from side to side. In a newborn, one can check for this by doing the rooting response. When the baby is hungry, his rooting response is vigorous and he will move his neck toward the side of the stimulus enabling one to check for the integrity of the sternocleidomastoid. In older children, one can check for this by having them turn their head from side to side. In young children, this can be done in response to a stimulus, e.g. a brightly colored object, if they are not able to do it voluntarily. Older children can voluntarily shrug their shoulders and check for the integrity of the trapezius muscle.

Hypoglossal

The twelfth cranial nerve controls the musculature of the tongue.[26] This muscle is important in the newborn since it is one muscle that is not covered by a large fat pad. One can look at the tongue to see if there are any abnormalities of muscle innervation reflected by muscle fasciculations.[29] To check for tongue function in the newborn, one can observe the baby when he cries to see if the tongue is symmetrical and midline. The rooting response can be stimulated in the inferior quadrant causing the baby to protrude his tongue. Older infants are difficult to assess for this except for simple observation of the tongue musculature as the child moves his tongue in his mouth. In older children voluntary tongue protrusion can be used.

Motor Exam

For the first clues in assessing the motor system of a child at any age we would start with the period of observation. This will give one early clues as to where to look for pathological findings. Although hypotonia and weakness are characteristic of lower motor neuron disease in the adult, these symptoms may result in disease of either the upper or the lower motor neurons in infants and young children.[29] Specifically, this means that a process involving the brain may cause weakness in the young child. Usually, in the adult, one sees this as a result of a problem either in the spinal cord or from the spinal cord to the muscle itself.

In the very immature where cooperation is limited, one must rely upon an examination of the special reflexes of infancy and childhood to determine whether there is dysfunction in the motor system. It is important to realize that development procedes in a bilaterally symmetrical fashion and that reflexes that are present on one side of the body should be present on the other. If this is not the case, there is a dysfunction on one or the other sides depending on the chronological age of the infant and which automatisms are present. Also, one would check for the persistence of certain pathological reflexes. When there is a developmental lag in the development of the gross motor system, there is usually a persistence of certain more primitive reflexes beyond the point one would expect their presence based on the child's chronological age.[31] In time, muscle groups may atrophy and certain muscles may become spastic (having greater resistance to passive motion). Since the approach to the examination of motor function depends upon the individual's chronological motor developmental age, the discussion of the motor exam will be divided into phases for the infant, the young child, and the older child.

Infant (birth to twenty-four months)

First one wants to get an impression of the body posture of the infant when lying supine. Is he lying in the infantile posture (predominant body posture from zero to four weeks of age, Figure 2)? In this posture, with the head in the midline, he would tend to lie with a very marked increase in his flexor tone in the arms and legs.[2] This can be appreciated by passively moving his extremities. At the age of four weeks to four months, the asymmetric tonic neck posture (Figure 3) becomes the predominant body posture.[30] This is elicited by turning the head to one side and checking for increase in extensor tone on the side to which the nose is pointing and increased flexor tone on the side to which the occiput is pointing.

It is often the hypertrophy of the infantile posture or occasionally the asymmetric tonic neck posture that leads to some of the postures peculiar to individuals with developmental delays in the area of their motor system. For example, someone who has not progressed out of the infantile period in terms of their gross motor function may persist in the infantile posture, at least in the upper extremities. They have a great increase in flexor tone and they maintain their hand in a flexed position and their thumb bent in toward the palm. This is often called the cortical thumb, but merely is a reflection of the persistence of the infantile posture that is a very primitive motor body posture. Eventually, the repetitive stimulation of the posture will lead to spasticity so that there would be a very marked increase in flexor tone when the infant has a persistence of the infantile posture.[32]

Although individual muscles cannot be accurately tested in the infant, large muscle groups can be adequately evaluated. This can be accomplished by the use of certain automatisms or basic body reflexes that are present in certain developmental stages. In addition to obtaining information concerning the child's muscle strength, one can also determine information concerning his developmental level (Table IV).

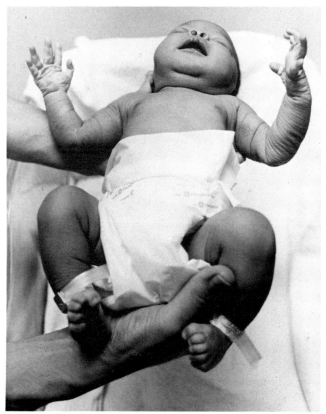

Figure 8. Moro reflex. When the infant is startled, he will extend both arms and gradually bring them toward the midline.

One reflex often tested in the infant is the Moro reflex, which is checked by startling the infant or by gently tilting the head up to 75° and then suddenly letting it fall down toward the table (Figure 8). When this is done, the infant will extend both of his arms in a symmetrical fashion and then gradually bring them in toward the midline. In addition, there is extension of the fingers at the point which the infant extends his arms. This reflex is present from birth until four months of age and begins to fade by four to five months.[32] This gives information concerning muscle strength at the shoulders, the elbows, and also the hands.

Another reflex that can be used is the traction grasp (Figure 9). To elicit this reflex, one puts stretch on the shoulder adductors and, when this is accomplished, the child will grasp down with his fingers.[2] This gives one the impression of shoulder girdle strength and tone as well as strength of the fingertips. The traction grasp can be facilitated by the use of a positive proprioceptive stimulus such as one's finger and then putting traction on shoulder adductors (Figure 10).[2] The infant will grasp down even harder with his fingers and one can actually pick a baby up from a surface by using the positive proprioceptive facilitation of the traction grasp. This reflex is normally present for the first four months of life and begins to fade by four to five months of age. It will give one information about strength at the shoulder girdle, the elbow, the wrist, and fingers.

The palmar grasp can be elicited by placing one's finger in a patient's palm and exerting pressure. When this is done, the reflex is for the infant to close his fingers tightly about the stimulus. This reflex is present from birth to four months of age.[2] At two months of age there is the development of the contact response (Figure 6).[8] If a stimulus is introduced into the proximal portion of the baby's palm and then gradually moved distally, as the stimulus arrives at the distal aspect of the hand, the baby will grasp his fingers down reflexly. This reflex is a way of determining strength at the fingertips.

The instinctive grasp is a response that begins to develop at five months of age (Figure 7). To elicit this response, one would gently stroke the medial or the lateral aspect of an infant's hand, and, at five months of age, he will orient his hand to the side of

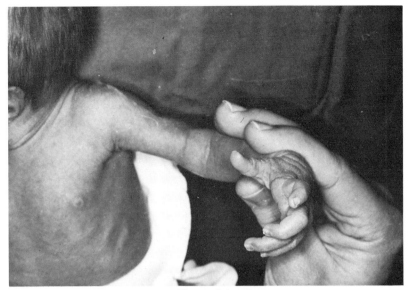

Figure 9A

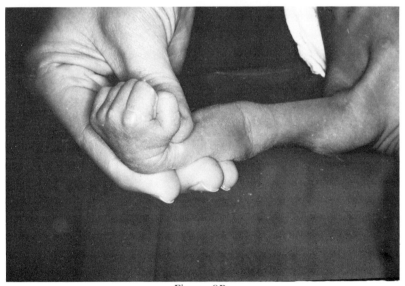

Figure 9B

Figure 9. The traction grasp. When stretch is placed upon the shoulder adductors as in 9A the infant will grasp down with his fingers as in 9B.

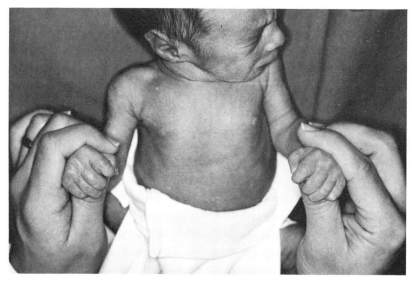

Figure 10A

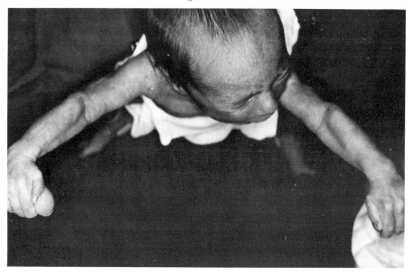

Figure 10B

Figure 10. Positive proprioceptive facilitation of the traction grasp. When stretch is placed on the shoulder adductors the use of a positive proprioceptive stimulus, e.g. the examiner's thumb, as in 10A will cause a facilitation of the traction grasp and enable the examiner to lift the infant by his exaggerated traction grasp as in 10B.

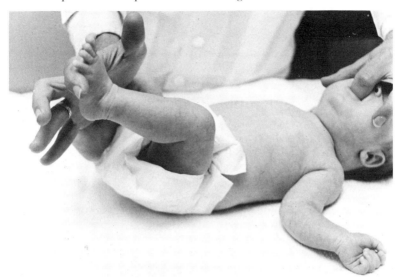

Figure 11A

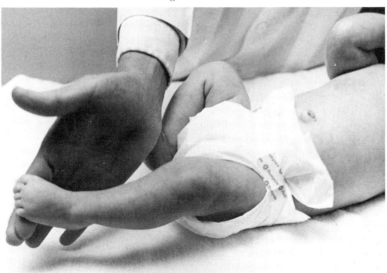

Figure 11B

Figure 11. Positive proprioceptive supporting response. Gentle pressure exerted on the ball of an infant's foot as in 11A will cause reflex extension at the hip, knee and ankle as in 11B.

the stimulus that is done totally independent of sight. Not only will he orient his hand to the side of the stimulus, but by eight to nine months of age he will grope out and grasp the stimulus totally independent of sight.[8]

There are several reflexes that can be checked in the lower extremities to aid in checking for muscle strength at various large muscle groups. The positive proprioceptive supporting response (Figure 11) is a response that is present in the newborn and indeed is persistent throughout one's life. To elicit this response, one puts gentle pressure on the ball of the infant's foot and when one does, the natural response is for the infant to extend his entire leg at the hip, the knee, and the ankle. In doing this one can get an impression of the strength of those large muscle groups.[34]

The plantar grasp (Figure 12) is elicited by placing a stimulus at the ball of the foot. The natural reflex response is for the infant to grasp his toes about the stimulus. This is present from birth until nine months of age[2] and is a way of checking for strength about the toes.

The infantile placing response is present at birth and can be elicited (Figure 4) by gently suspending the infant in the air and touching the anterior aspect of his foot to a surface. The response is for him to flex his hip, knee and ankle and then gradually extend his leg at the hip, the knee, and the ankle and place it flat upon the surface.[6] The placing response becomes more sophisticated at four months of age. The four month old, when he is suspended in air and the anterior aspect of his foot is touched to a surface, will grope out after the shape of the surface until he reaches to the top (Figure 5). This occurs with medial and lateral stimulation of the infant's foot at six months of age and would occur at nine months of age with stimulation of the posterior aspect of an infant's foot.[7, 34]

In the six month old, one can check for the lateral propping response (Figure 13), where if one tilts the sitting baby to one side, the natural reflex is for him to extend the arm on the side to which he is being tilted.[31] This special reflex is useful in assessing the infant's muscle strength and tone at the shoulder, elbow, wrist and hand.

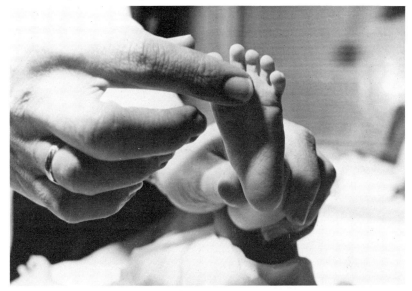

Figure 12A

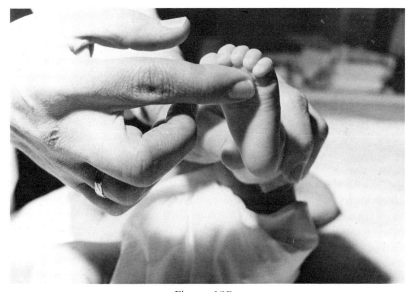

Figure 12B

Figure 12. Plantar grasp. A stimulus to the ball of the foot as in 12A will cause reflex plantar flexion of the toes about the stimulus as in 12B.

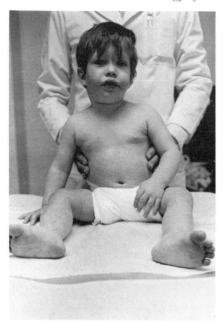 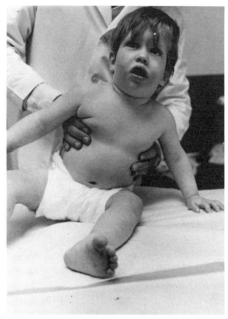

Figure 13. The lateral propping response. When the infant is seated as in 13A and tilted laterally he will extend his arm toward the surface as in 13B.

The deep tendon reflexes of infants may also show some regional differences.[35] For example, from birth to the first four weeks of age, the triceps jerk may not be elicited because of the very predominant flexor tone in the upper extremities seen with the infantile posture. Also, the ankle jerk may not be present because of the very marked dorsiflexor tone present at the ankle. By four to six weeks of age, all the deep tendon reflexes should be present. In addition, there are some normal newborns who have ankle clonus (up to 12 beats), which is not necessarily associated with pathology. It is definitely abnormal to see knee clonus or clonus in other areas. The plantar response (Babinski test) is variable for the first year of life and should become flexor after twelve months of age.[36, 37] This response is elicited by the introduction of a noxious distally moving stimulus, starting at the base of the foot and gradually moving toward the ball of the foot.[38]

Older Infant and Young Child

The older infant and young child can carry out a number of movements, e.g. reaching for colorful objects, sitting, crawling, and walking. All these movements allow one to assess motor function by mere observation. The deep tendon reflexes should all be present by four weeks of age.[35] Usually, those in the upper extremities are slightly less active than those in the lower extremities. Ankle clonus is never normal in an older infant or child. The plantar response is clearly flexor.[37]

Unfortunately, it is still not possible to do individual muscle group testing in this age bracket. Yet, one can test the function of large muscle groups by other basic body reflexes. One such reflex for checking muscle strength in the upper extremity is the parachute and wheelbarrow response. In the parachute response (Figure 14), the infant is held in air in the prone position and thrust forward toward a firm surface. The normal response of the infant is to extend his arms flatly to the surface. It is from the parachute response that a wheelbarrow maneuver (Figure 15) can be tested once the infant is supporting his own weight upon outstretched arms. He can be induced to hand walk alternating arms by gently pushing his body forward.[31]

Much information concerning the function of the lower extremities can be gained by watching the child walk and climb upstairs. This is often useful in assessing the strength at the hip girdle as well as the knee. At four years of age, one can have a child do a sit-up, which he should be able to accomplish without assistance as another means of checking for strength at the hip girdle. Another simple test of hip function and muscle strength of the lower extremities is to have the child rise to a standing position from a prone position on the floor without touching anything in the room. If he is not able to do this without leaning on his own knees and literally climbing with his hands on his upper legs for assistance to attain the erect posture, it is called the Gower's sign. The Gower's sign is an indicator of hip weakness.

Observation of the child's walking and running can be extremely useful to determine the presence of hip or leg problems.

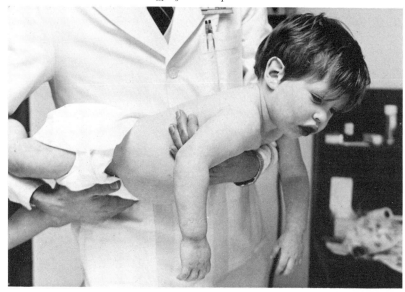

Figure 14A

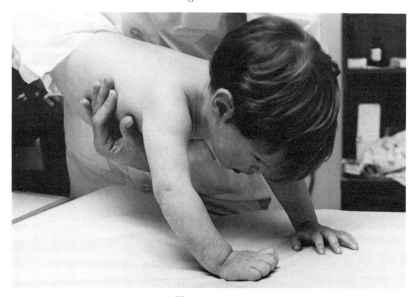

Figure 14B

Figure 14. The parachute response. When the infant is suspended in the prone position as in 14A and thrust forward toward a firm surface, he will reflexly extend his arm as in 14B.

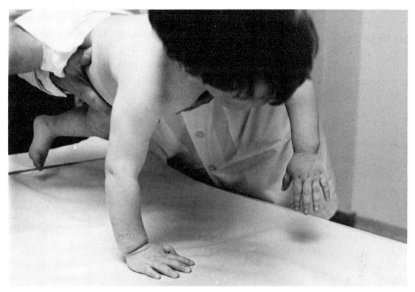

Figure 15. The wheelbarrow response. When the infant in 14B has his weight supported by outstretched arms, he can be induced to alternate arms in a crawl by gently pushing his body forward.

One would be looking for deviations of the feet, whether or not there is a waddling gait, whether or not there is some circumduction of one leg, and whether there is a wide-based gait. One also would look for any normal associated movements or peculiar posturings of the arms as the child walks.

Older Child

After the age of four to five years, one can perform individual muscle group testing. It is possible to check individual muscles by having the child push against the examiner in a variety of maneuvers to test specific muscle function. Still much information can be gained by good observation of children in this age bracket. Information can be obtained by having them heel walk or toe walk where one would be looking for exaggeration of primitive postures or exaggeration of abnormalities of gait. These maneuvers often assist one in determining some of the soft neurological signs. Individual muscle strength really can be graded on a scale of 0 to 5, 0 having no muscle contraction whatsoever upon volition and 5 having maximum resistance to passive motion.[31]

Fine Motor Examination

Just as there is normal progression of the acquisition of gross motor skills there is a normal progression of fine motor skills. The quality of a child's fine motor skills can be checked during the examination using the schema outlined in Table II. This schema gives one a concrete measure of the individual's fine motor performance based on his chronological age.[8, 9]

Sensory Exam

The quality of the sensory exam depends upon the developmental level of the child being tested. The infant is especially difficult to evaluate because all but the most punitive sensory exams require cooperation. In infants, there are some reflexes that could be used to check for sensory modalities. For example, the rooting response is a cutaneous sensory response so that, if one is able to perform the rooting response, one knows that the infant is able to perceive sensations about the mouth. Also, in the hand or in the foot, one can check for the avoiding response. This is present normally from birth to four months of age and is elicited (Figure 16) by gently stroking the posterior aspect or lateral aspect of an infant's hand or his foot.[39] The natural response would be for him to open his fingers out or fan out his toes. This reflex is a means of evaluation of the infant's ability to perceive light touch. At a later stage of development, one could check for the instinctive grasping response, which is also a cutaneous response that relies upon light touch. This response becomes apparent at five months of age and becomes fully developed by nine months (Figure 7).

The testing of pain stimuli in an infant is very difficult. One needs to get the infant at rest, introduce the noxious stimulus into an area where he can perceive pain, quiet the infant down, and then gradually move the stimulus toward the areas in question. Each time the stimulus is introduced, the infant must be quieted down and then restimulated.

In order to accomplish an accurate exam of more sophisti-

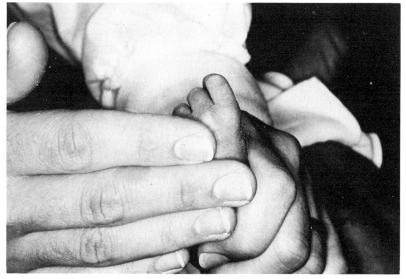

Figure 16A

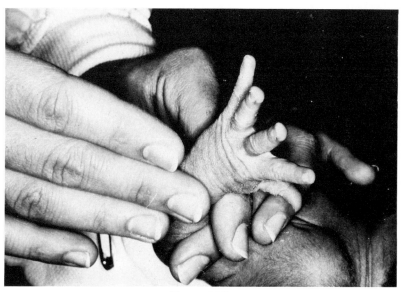

Figure 16B

Figure 16. The avoiding response. Gentle cutaneous touch to an infant's hand as in 16A will cause him to reflexly fan out his fingers as in 16B.

cated modalities one must rely on patient cooperation. Unfortunately this is exceedingly difficult to perform before the chronological age of five years. The sensory modalities that can be tested include light touch, pain, vibratory sensation, position sensation, graphesthesia, two point discrimination, and stereognosis.[40]

Coordination

Unfortunately this modality cannot be checked until the infant is able to reach for objects (six months). Certainly when one is dealing with an older child (three to five years) one can elicit cooperation to do finger to nose testing or imitation or rapidly alternating movements. Certain maneuvers can yield the desired information in the first year of life. After six months of age, the child can reach for objects laterally.[3] One can see if the movement is accomplished smoothly and accomplished with equal facility on the left and on the right. By the age of nine to eleven months, the infant is reaching for pellets. The infant's ability to smoothly reach toward the pellet and grasp it with a pincer grasp can be studied. By fifteen months of age, the infant is capable of grasping a pellet with a pincer grasp and then releasing it into a container upon command or imitation.[3] The integrity of this motion can be studied to determine whether or not there is any evidence of incoordination. This is a very good test of coordination up until three to five years of age, after which finger to nose testing can be used. Accurate finger to nose, heel to shin, and rapidly alternating movement testing[40] is not accomplished until the child is past five years of age in his fine motor coordinative skills.

Gait and Station

Again observation is exceptionally important in evaluating the child's gait and station. One would observe how a child stands at rest, how he moves, and how he walks. Are toes pointed in? Are toes pointed out? Is the gait wide based? Is the gait wide based as a toddler gait of twelve to twenty-four months, or is it the normal stance with the toes pointed directly ahead as a child who is three years of age or older?[41] It is interesting to note that children who have been hypotonic tend to maintain a wide-based toeing-out gait for a longer period of time than is normal. In addition, children who have had a developmental lag and have not acquired the walking skill until greater than eighteen months will persist with a slightly wide-based gait beyond the normal period unless spasticity is also present.

The child's regular gait should be observed as well as his heel and toe walking.[22] This can give information about the strength of the muscles about the ankle and information concerning soft neurological signs. Heel and toe walking stress the nervous system and tend to exaggerate soft neurological signs if they are present. For example, if one has a child below the age of five years heel walk or toe walk, it is not uncommon for them to posture both of their arms in the infantile posture (Figure 2). After five years of age this should no longer be present. If it is present bilaterally or unilaterally, it is a soft neurological sign of subtle nervous system dysfunction.

The Head

Much attention should be paid to the head of a child with a developmental disability. The head circumference should be measured and compared to norms based on age and sex.[42] It should be determined if the child's head is too large or too small for his age. In addition, one would look for any scars or abnormality of closure of the sutures and anterior or posterior fontanelles. The posterior fontanelle closes by six to eight weeks and the anterior fontanelle closes by sixteen to eighteen months.[43] In infants, a transillumination maneuver should be performed in which a flashlight with a rubber-tipped applicator is moved over a child's head in a dark room. This is done to look for areas of increased or decreased illumination.[44] Transillumination can be performed in a normally lit room with a Chun-gun (a specialized light for transillumination).[45]

Table IV
DEVELOPMENTAL TESTING SCHEMA — BIRTH TO TWELVE YEARS

Birth to One Month

I. Head Function.
 Eye following: fix and follow 90° from midline.
 Rooting: all four quadrants.
 Sucking: strong.
II. Hand function.
 Hand avoiding.
 Palmar grasp.
 Traction grasp and positive proprioceptive facilitation of traction grasp.
III. Foot and leg function.
 Positive proprioceptive supporting.
 Foot avoiding.
 Plantar grasp.
 Neonatal placing and stepping.
IV. General body.
 Infantile posture.
 Moro reflex.
 Sitting: marked kyphosis.
 Prone: head side to side and face just off bed.
 Arm traction for head support: marked head lag.
V. Reflexes.
 May have no ankle or triceps DTRs.
 Plantar response: variable.

One Month to Two Months

I. Head function.
 Eye following: 135° and crossed midline.
 Rooting: all four quadrants.
 Sucking: strong.
II. Hand function.
 Hand avoiding.
 Palmar grasp.
 Traction grasp and positive proprioceptive facilitation.
III. Foot and leg function.
 Positive proprioceptive supporting.
 Foot avoiding.
 Plantar grasp.
 Neonatal placing and stepping.
IV. General body.
 Asymmetric tonic neck posture.
 Moro reflex.
 Sitting: moderate kyphosis.
 Prone: head side to side, face just off bed.
 Arm traction: lag with some dorsiflexion.
V. Reflexes.
 All DTRs present.
 Plantar: variable.

Two to Four Months

I. Head function.
 Eye following: 180°.
 Rooting: all four quadrants.
 Sucking: strong.

Table IV — *Continued*

II. Hand function.
    Hand avoiding.
    Palmar grasp.
    Traction grasp and positive proprioceptive facilitation.
    Contact grasp.
III. Foot and leg function.
    Positive proprioceptive supporting.
    Foot avoiding.
    Plantar grasp.
    Neonatal placing and stepping.
IV. General body.
    Asymmetric tonic neck.
    Moro reflex.
    Sitting: moderate kyphosis, slight head extension.
    Prone: head and face 45° to bed and legs straight.
    Arm traction for head support: head level.
V. Reflexes.
    All deep tendon reflexes are present.
    Plantar: variable.

Four to Five Months

I. Head function.
    Eye following: full range.
    Rooting: fading in awakened state and present when drowsy.
II. Hand function.
    Traction grasp: fading.
    Hand avoiding: fading.
    Palmar grasp: fading.
    Contact grasp: fading.
    Orientation phase of instinctive grasp: beginning.
III. Foot and leg function.
    Positive proprioceptive supporting.
    Plantar grasp.
    Foot avoiding: fading.
    Placing and stepping: fading.
    True anterior placing.
IV. General body.
    Asymmetric tonic neck: fading.
    Moro reflex.
    Sitting: sits in frog position up to ten seconds.
    Prone: head 90° to bed, support on arms.
    Rolls over: prone to supine and supine to prone.
V. Reflexes.
    Plantar: flexor.

Five to Seven Months

I. Head function.
    Rooting: drowsy only.
II. Hand function.
    Traction grasp: gone.
    Hand avoiding: gone.
    Palmar grasp: gone.
    Contact grasp: gone.
    Orientation and groping to instinctive grasp.
    Reaches with full fisted grasp.

Table IV — *Continued*

III. Foot function.
    Positive proprioceptive supporting.
    Plantar grasp: gone.
    Foot avoiding: gone.
    Placing and stepping: gone.
    True anterior, medial, and lateral placing.
IV. General body.
    Asymmetrical tonic neck and Moro: gone.
    Sitting: unsupported when placed.

Seven to Nine Months

  I. Head function.
    Rooting is fading in drowsiness and gone by nine months.
 II. Hand function.
    Orientation, groping and grasp to instinctive grasp.
    Grasp changing to thumb and three fingers.
    Will transfer hand to hand and hand to mouth.
III. Foot function.
    Positive proprioceptive supporting.
    Plantar grasp: fading and gone.
    True anterior, medial, and lateral placing.
    Posterior placing beginning.
IV. General body.
    Begins to sit alone.
  V. Speech.
    Begins to use repetitive syllables.

Nine to Twelve Months

  I. Head function.
    Rooting gone.
 II. Hand function.
    Instinctive grasp fully developed.
    Pincer grasp and reaches for pellets.
III. Foot function.
    Anterior, medial, lateral, and posterior placing.
IV. General body.
    Stands and walks holding on.
  V. Speech.
    Uses repetitive syllables with meaning.

Twelve to Eighteen Months

  I. Head function.
    Will have smooth eye tracking by eighteen months.
 II. Hand function.
    Reaches for pellets with pincer grasp.
    Will place one marble in container: fifteen months.
    Will place three marbles in container: seventeen months.
    Will place three marbles in container with cap: eighteen months.
III. General body.
    Walks alone by eighteen months.
IV. Speech.
    Will use single words by eighteen months.

Table IV — *Continued*

Eighteen to Twenty-Four Months

I. Hand function.
Will build a five block tower: eighteen to twenty-one months.
Will build a six to seven block tower: twenty-one to twenty-four months.
Will scribble with crayon.
Classical figures of Gesell: three on one card.*
II. General body.
Physiologically ready for bowel and bladder training.
III. Speech.
Will use phrases by twenty-four months.

Twenty-Four to Thirty-Six Months

I. Hand function.
Places classical figures of Gesell one per card and inappropriately: twenty-four to thirty months.
Places classical figures of Gesell one per card and appropriately: thirty to thirty-six months.
Will draw a circle.
II. Speech: Gesell pictures.†
Names three and identifies five: twenty-four months.
Names five and identifies seven: thirty months.
Names eight and identifies ten: thirty-six months.

Three to Four Years

I. Hand function.
Will draw + and X.
II. Speech function: Gesell pictures.
Will name eight and identify ten: thirty-six months.
Will name ten and identify ten: forty-two months.
Will make labial, lingual, and gutteral sounds.

Four to Five Years

I. Hand function.
Draws a square with rounded corners.
Begins to place French curve.
II. Fine motor function.
Begins to disassociate head from eye movement.

Five to Six Years

I. Hand function.
Draws a square and a triangle.
Can place French curve.

---

* The classical figures of Gesell consist of a circle, square, and triangle and their forms.

† The Gesell pictures consist of ten items (dog, house, shoe, leaf, basket, clock, stars, book, flag and cup) that are first individually presented to child to name and then placed upon a flat surface and the child is asked to point to each item as it is named.

Table IV — *Continued*

II. Fine motor function.
    Can do rapid alternating movements with arm extended.
    Can do serial opposition of fingers.
    Can do heel and shin movement.
    Can do heel tapping.
    Can hop on each foot.

Six to Seven Years

  I. Hand function.
     Can draw a longitudinal and vertical diamond.
 II. Fine motor function.
     Can carry out rapid fire commands.
III. Reading.‡
     First grade materials.

Seven to Eight Years

  I. Hand function.
     Draws a union jack and diamond in a square.
 II. Fine motor function.
     Can do cheek filling and alternate cheek filling.
     Can do fine facial movement.
     Has right and left orientation.
III. Reading.‡
     Reads second grade material.
     No longer has letter reversal or mirror reading.

Eight to Nine Years

  I. Hand function.
     Draws a four-pointed star.
 II. Fine motor function.
     Fine lingual movements.
III. Reading.‡
     Reads third grade material.

Nine to Twelve Years

  I. Hand function.
     Draws a three dimensional cube.
 II. Reading.‡
     Fourth grade: nine to ten years.
     Fifth grade: ten to eleven years.
     Sixth grade: eleven to twelve years.

‡ Gilmore Oral Reading Test

Chapter 3

NORMAL EMBRYOLOGY OF THE CENTRAL NERVOUS SYSTEM AND ITS RELATIONSHIP TO THE OCCURRENCE OF CONGENITAL MALFORMATIONS

C ONGENITAL MALFORMATIONS are structural defects that are present at the time of birth. Because of the anatomical nature of the central nervous system (enclosed in a bony cavity) and because of its functional immaturity at birth; many central nervous system malformations may not be noted until beyond the neonatal period. Malformations are observed in the neonate if they involve the bony coverings of the skull or spine or if they involve the face.

The types of deficits that are seen may be the result of several different processes.[46] There may be a failure of structures to fuse or come together. This is seen in the production of spina bifida, encephaloceles or meningomyeloceles. There may be a defect in the normal cleavage of structures that could result in median cleft syndromes, which is, in the most severe case, a cyclops. There may be a failure of the cell population to migrate to its usual location. This is etiologic in producing cortical heterotopias. There may be a defect in cellular differentiation, which could lead to the absence of various structures or to the persistence of certain immature cell populations resulting in congenital rest, which may subsequently lead to neoplastic processes such as hamartomas.

In the nongenetically determined malformation, the timing of the insult relative to the stage of embryonal development is of critical importance, since the embryo is differentially susceptible to teratogenic agents at different stages in development.[47, 48] The well-known example of this phenomena is the rubella virus,[49] which, when it attacks the fetus in the first trimester, produces a characteristic pattern of anomalies, but, if the fetus is

47

infected late in the third trimester, there may be minimal or no effect.

When an embryo is exposed to a teratogen early in embryogenesis there may be embryonal death. When a teratogenic agent occurs at the stage of organ differentiation, several malformations may be produced. The type of malformation depends not only upon the type of teratogen, but also upon the timing of the injury relative to the type of developmental processes occurring.[50] During the third trimester (period of organ growth), fetal susceptibility to teratogenic agents decreases, and their effect may be inhibition of growth or degeneration of existing tissue. The genotype of the embryo may also influence the effect of a teratogenic agent.[51] This has been shown in animal experiments where different strains of the same species have different susceptibilities to the same teratogenic agent.[52] Teratogenic agents may also be highly specific for certain cell populations.[53] This is seen with the rubella virus that specifically attacks the developing nervous system and the developing cardiac system.[54] Many teratogens have organ specificity and do not produce multisystemic abnormalities.

Malformations may be the result of environmental teratogens or the result of intrinsic factors.[46] There are several environmental factors that are known to cause malformations in the central nervous system of the fetus. Hypoxia is a common cause of such conditions. Hypoxia can arise from any situation that would cause the fetus to have decreased amounts of oxygen during development, focally or generally.[55] Conditions such as placental separation (abruptio) and bleeding may lead to fetal hypoxia. Another factor that may come into play is placental insufficiency (where the fetus does not get sufficient blood and oxygen for its normal growth).[56, 57]

Infectious agents are well known teratogens to the central nervous system. Viral infections such as rubella and cytomegalic inclusion virus are known to produce characteristic patterns of malformation.[58] In addition, protozoans such as toxoplasmosis and bacteria such as syphilis are also infectious teratogenic agents for the fetus.[59]

Radiation in significant amounts can produce malformations

of the developing brain.[60-62] This was borne out with the effects on the fetuses that were exposed to radiation from the atomic bomb explosion on Hiroshima. The critical factors in determining the severity of the insult were the distance from the center of the explosion and the time in gestation that exposure occurred. Those exposed very early in gestation (the first trimester) were at considerable risk for developing central nervous system malformation, whereas those exposed during the last trimester were at minimal risk. Those exposed with high intensity (close to the center of the explosion) were more severely affected than those exposed more distal to the explosion's center.[63, 64]

There have been numerous animal experiments involving radiation to the embryo demonstrating defects in neurogenesis or defects in cellular interconnections in the nervous system (within the arborization of the dentritic tree). The findings correlated with the amount of radiation and the timing of the radiation insult in gestation.

Hormonal factors may play a role in producing defects in neurogenesis.[65, 66] The most well studied is the thyroid hormone whose deficiency is known to produce cretinism.[67-70]

Nutritional deficiencies are an often erroneously incriminated etiology of fetal malformation.[71] In order for defective nutrition to be etiologic in producing malformations, the deficiency must be very severe since the fetus will preferentially utilize glucose and oxygen at the expense of the mother.

The intrinsic factors etiologic in producing congenital malformations are chromosomal and genetic.[46] It is well known that there are several chromosomal deficiencies such as Trisomy 21, Trisomy 13, and Trisomy 15, which produce very characteristic patterns of anomalies involving many parts of the body as well as the central nervous system. Chromosomal difficulties affecting the nervous system may result from either the deletion of chromosomal materials such as the 4p− syndrome or by the presence of additional malformed chromosomes such as in the Trisomy 21 syndrome.[72] Chromosomal abnormalities can be detected by the performance of chromosomal analysis upon the white blood cells or upon other cultured cells, e.g. fibroblasts from the skin, in the affected child. Amniocentesis may be performed during pregnancy and cells cultured for chromosomal analysis.[72] This is often done in women who have late life pregnancies where the incidence of Trisomy 21 (Down's syndrome) is increased.[74]

Genetic factors that may cause congenital anomalies are often more difficult to discern, primarily because there are no demonstrable markers with our current state of knowledge. Clinical patterns of genetic abnormalities may be quite specific and lead to a diagnosis.[72] Conditions such as Meckel's syndrome[75] and Robert's syndrome[76] are autosomal recessive conditions that may lead to structural abnormalities in the central nervous system. It is important to diagnose these conditions because of their genetic basis and the possibility of their recurrence in future pregnancies within the same family.[77]

Genetic abnormalities may be a more frequent cause of malformations of the central nervous system than previously considered. This has been shown with neural tube defects, e.g. meningomyelocele and encephalocele. In a study of infants with neural tube defects who were examined at postmortem, it was found that 12 percent had their defect as a result of a genetic or chromosomal abnormality. In many cases, this had been undetected prior to the postmortem examination.[77] The families of children with these genetic defects should be aware of the genetic basis of the defect, since there is a method of intrauterine diagnosis of neural tube defects by alphafetoprotein determination. A rise in alphafetoprotein is a sign of a neural tube defect that is open to the aminotic fluid.[78] In these cases, the mother would have the opportunity for a therapeutic abortion.

A knowledge of the normal development of the central nervous system during embryogenesis is important to the understanding of the etiologic factors producing malformations. The nervous system begins in the third week of embryogenesis from a thin plate of ectoderm (Figure 17). Within a few days, the neural plate begins to fold in the midline and forms a neural groove. The edges about the groove begin to fuse within this third week of gestation. The fusion of the tube begins in the region of the fourth somite. Fusion progresses both cephalad and caudally. The areas that will be the cranial and caudal ends

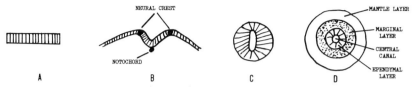

Figure 17. Embryonic development of the neural tube. The nervous system develops from a thin plate of ectoderm (A); which folds (B); and fuses to form the neural tube (C). The neural tube becomes differentiated in several layers (D).

of the nervous system fuse last, initially remaining open to the amnionic cavity (Figure 18a). By the twenty-third day of embryogenesis, the anterior end has closed, and, by the twenty-fifth day of embryogenesis, the posterior end has closed. At the end of the fourth week, the central nervous system is an enclosed tube (Figure 17c) with overlying ectoderm, no longer in communication with the amnionic cavity.[46]

If there is a defect in embryogenesis or the introduction of a neurotoxic teratogenic agent at this point in gestation, the result may be a persistent opening in the tube (Figure 18a). Should the opening occur at the posterior (caudal) end of the tube, the result is a form of spina bifida. This may vary from spina bifida occulta, which would simply be a defect in the bony structure about the caudal end of the spine, to a defect that involves the

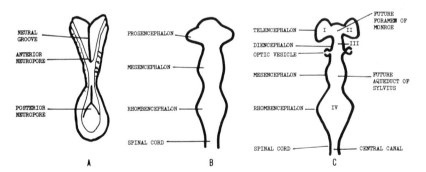

Figure 18. Fusion and differentiation of the primitive neural tube. The neural tube begins to fuse within the first three weeks of embryogenesis (A); then differentiates into specialized structures (B and C) that will mature into the human nervous system. (Roman numerals refer to the ventricular system.)

spinal cord, the bony spine, and skin covering the spinal cord, which would be a meningomyelocele.[79, 80] If the insult were to occur at the twenty-third day, the defect may involve the cephalad (anterior) end of the neural tube. The defects produced would range from meningoceles where the cranium fails to fuse, to meningoencephaloceles where the meninges and cranial contents are external to the skull, to no development of the cranial end of the neural tube producing anencephaly.[81, 82]

During the fourth week of embryogenesis, the neural tube undergoes several other changes. There are bends in the tube. The cephalic end undergoes cellular proliferation and dilatation, which differentiates the cephalic end of the tube into areas destined to become the prosencephalon (the forebrain), the mesencephalon (the midbrain), and the rhombencephalon (the hindbrain) (Figure 18b).

Flexures occur in two places. The cephalic flexure occurs between the rhombencephalon and the mesencephalon. The cervical flexure occurs between what will be the end of the hindbrain and the spinal cord. If there is a defect in the bending of the tube at this point, the contents that would normally be found in the posterior fossa of the skull would lie in the cervical area of the spinal cord. This is what is seen in the Arnold-Chiari malformation, where portions of the medulla and/or cerebellum are found to lie in the cervical cord rather than in their normal location, the posterior fossa. If this is very pronounced, portions of the fourth ventricle may be misplaced into the cervical spine and result in hydrocephalus. The Arnold-Chiari malformation is frequently seen with meningomyelocele since the cervical flexuring of the tube occurs at approximately the same point in the embryogenesis as the closure of the caudal and the neural tube.[46]

Further differentiation of the anterior aspect of the neural tube occurs during the fifth week. The prosencephalon differentiates into an anterior portion (telencephalon) with two bulges for the cerebral hemispheres and a posterior portion (diencephalon) where the optic vesicles begin to form (Figure 18c). The optic vesicles and, subsequently, the optic nerves and eyes are really specialized neuronal elements.[46] Processes that will affect the central nervous system are also capable of affecting the optic nerves and retina. Disease processes such as intrauterine acquired infections that affect the brain may also produce effects in the eye.[84] One may look at the retina and eye for manifestations of the insult, e.g. chorioretinitis. Processes producing malformations of the brain during embryogenesis may also produce abnormalities of ocular embryogenesis. An example of this would be arhinencephaly where optic defects and intracranial defects coexist.[85] Disease processes occurring later in life such as neuronal storage diseases, e.g. Tay-Sachs, will produce changes in the retina as well as in the brain.[86] Diseases in the adult such as multiple sclerosis often affect the retina as well as the brain.[87] The common embryogenic origin of the brain and the eye is another reason why a good neurological examination involves good funduscopic examination.

During the fifth week, the mesencephalon differentiates into the midbrain and the rhombencephalon differentiates into an anterior portion (metencephalon), which will become the pons and cerebellum, and a posterior portion (myelencephalon), which will become the medulla.[46]

By the middle of the fourth week, the cells of the neural tube have differentiated into three layers (Figure 17d). The innermost layer is the ependymal layer that surrounds a central hollow core. Adjacent to the ependymal layer is a mantle (germinal) layer that consists of neuroblasts. The outer portion is the marginal layer that consists of nerve fibers from the neurons of the mantle layer and would subsequently become the white matter. The center of the neural tube is a hollow area that, in the anterior aspect, will differentiate into the ventricular system. In the caudal aspect, this will become the central core of the spinal cord.

In the spinal cord and lower medulla, the developmental pattern maintains the anatomy of an internal neuronal layer and an external fiber (white matter) layer. As the germinal cells differentiate, the dorsal cells of the tube will differentiate into sensory cells and the ventral cells into motor cells. This differentiation of the mantle layer produces an alar (sensory) plate and a basilar (motor) plate. There is a small indentation between these areas known as the sulcus limitans. This separation produces an anterior horn cell area (ventral) in the spinal cord, which controls the motor aspect of the spinal cord, and a posterior horn (dorsal), which controls the sensory aspect of the spinal cord. This relationship between the motor and sensory neurons exists throughout the rhombencephalon, but overgrowth of other structures, such as the fourth ventricle, will distort this relationship and alter the gross anatomy of the developing tube to that seen in the mature brain stem.[46]

At thirty weeks of age, the spinal cord and the spinal column are aligned. By the time the infant is born, the spinal cord ends between the second and third vertebrae. In the adult, the spinal cord ends between the first and second lumbar vertebrae. The alteration in the anatomical relationship between the spinal cord and spinal column correlates with the growth of the bones of the spinal column.[46] It is the differential in length of the spinal cord and spinal column that enables physicians to safely sample CSF by lumbar tap (spinal tap).

By the middle of the fourth to fifth week, the mantle layer germinal cells in the telencephalon create neurons that migrate through the marginal layer to the surface of the modified neural tube. These cells will become the neurons of the mature cerebral cortex, forming an outer layer of gray matter and an inner layer of white matter (neuronal cell processes). This is in contradistinction to the spinal cord where the neurons remain in the area of the mantle layer or germinal layer and their cell processes remain in the marginal layer (outer white matter). In the telencephalon, the neurons are continually made until the twenty-fourth week of gestation. All the neurons that are present in the mature cerebral hemisphere will have been formed and/or started their migration to the surface. (No cortical neurons will be formed after the twenty-fourth week of gestation.) The germinal elements in the mantle layer will continue to produce glial cells until two to four weeks after birth.[88]

Should there be some defect in the normal neuronal migration and the neurons do not migrate completely to the surface, cortical heterotopias are produced.[89] These are islands of neurons within white matter of cerebral hemispheres. This is a defect that is occasionally seen in the developmentally disabled. In normal individuals, small cortical heterotopias occasionally may be found. Once the cells reach the surface of the telencephalon there is a rapid proliferation of cell processes. As more cells arrive at the surface and the cell processes proliferate there is an overgrowth of this area causing it to bend and form what are called gyri or hills, which become separated by sulci or valleys. Thus, the normal six layered neuronal pattern of the cerebral hemisphere is formed. At twenty-four weeks, when the first sulcus appears and with further development other sulci appear, if the migratory pattern is abnormal, abnormal gyral and sulcal patterns may be produced. This is seen in conditions such as lissencephaly (lack of gyri) or focal or diffuse polymicrogyri (multiple small gyri and sulci).[89]

The most important factor in embryology of the central nervous system is that the nervous system begins developing very early in gestation and the cortical neuronal cells are completely formed by twenty-four weeks of gestation. The only remaining cells formed in the cortex are the glial cells, which continue to form until shortly after birth. Teratogenic agents, which can affect the organogenesis of the nervous system, must have had their effect before twenty-four weeks of gestation. Teratogenic agents may exert effects later, but the effects are on the formed cell population rather than on structural organ defects within the nervous system.[50]

For the explanation of nongenetically determined malformations of the central nervous system, much attention has been focused on the effects of viral infections upon the developing nervous system. Animal experiments in embryogenesis have produced defects that are analogous to defects seen in human central nervous system embryogenesis.[53] Most people are familiar with the effect of viral infections on developing fetuses that may result in abnormalities of the brain, e.g. rubella and cytomegalic inclusion virus.[49, 54] Pathologic changes found in the central nervous system following these infections may include encephalomalacia, calcifications and signs of chronic inflammation. In addition, there may be some signs of immunological contact with the virus by elevations of viral antibody titers in the serum of the newborn infant. These changes have been regarded as signs of antecedent or chronic viral infections of the immature brain.

A series of studies in laboratory animals have shown that viral infections during early embryogenesis induce sequelae that resemble primary defects seen in human neuroembryogenesis. The defects neuropathologically appear noninflammatory and lack signs suggesting antecedent infection, including a lack of an elevation in antibody titers to the specific viral agent. These malformations resemble malformations of the brain previously felt to be of toxic, genetic, or vascular etiology.[53]

If chick embryos are inoculated at twenty-four hours of age with live influenza A virus, certain developmental anomalies result that are limited to the neural tube.[80, 81] These defects include a defect in the normal neural tube cervical flexure, a collapse of the primitive brain, and a failure of closure of the caudal spinal area. The congenital anomalies were seen only after inoculation with active live virus. They were only induced in some of the embryos. Some embryos did not survive the infection and would represent abortions. In the survivors, defects of meningomyelocele and Arnold-Chiari malformation were produced. The failure of their neural tube to close (meningomyelocele) was not associated with the necrosis of cells at the neural tube area and mitotic activity of the cells appeared quite normal. There were no inflammatory cells in this area. By the time the chick was born there was no evidence of an infection having occurred in his neural tube. The defects were analogous to those seen in children afflicted with meningomyelocele and Arnold-Chiari malformation.

Experiments with the bluetongue virus of sheep have been used to show the potential effects of viral infections on various stages in neuroembryogenesis.[90, 91] Animals were sacrificed at different times after their infection. When bluetongue virus is introduced into the fetuses of pregnant ewes at various stages of development and the animal is sacrificed within 6 to 100 days after inoculation, different effects were seen depending upon the timing of the infection. Ewes inoculated between fifty and fifty-five days of gestation produced lambs with hydranencephaly. In these lambs, there was focal necrosis in the subependymal zones by the twenty-first day after infection and this involved all developing cells in the cerebral hemisphere except the ependymal cells. Initially, all undifferentiated cells including potential neuroblasts and neuroglioblasts in the subependymal ventricular zone were affected. Loss of these cells resulted in total absence of formation of the cerebral cortex. Necrosis also included the undifferentiated cells of the metencephalon and the retina. In the retina this lead to extensive retinal damage and retinal dysplasia. This produced anomaly is analogous to the anomaly of hydranencephaly seen in the human where there is a lack of cortex and dysplasia of the optic nerve and retina.

The fetal lambs that were inoculated at seventy-five to seventy-eight days of gestation showed porencephalic cysts (cysts within the cerebral hemisphere that communicate with the ventricular system). Pseudoporencephalic cysts are often mistakenly labeled as porencephalic cysts. (Pseudoporencephalic cysts do not communicate with the ventricular system). In these lambs, the porencephalic cystic cavities were localized largely in the white matter. Early changes were focal vacuolated areas in the subcortical white matter. Focal necrosis occurred in the subependymal zone leading to the porencephalic cysts. This is analogous to the porencephalic cysts that are seen in humans. In some animals, hypoplasia was seen in areas of the cerebellum.

In the fetal lambs that were inoculated after one hundred days of gestation, the only finding was evidence of chronic inflammatory reaction manifested by subependymal glial nodules. This subependymal reactive process was observed without evidence of vasculitis or vascular necrosis.

In the bluetongue virus study, there was no evidence of infection of the vascular endothelium but extensive infection was localized to the germinal cells of the telencephalon. It is this cell population lying adjacent to the embryonal ventricle that contains the neuroblasts and glioblasts. If this infection occurs in the first trimester, the undifferentiated germinal cell population is large, and infection produced massive necrosis and cavitation of the cerebral hemispheres (hydranencephaly). By midgestation most of the cortical plate neurons have developed but there are still areas of germinal cell proliferation. Infections of these germinal cells lead to focal areas of encephalomalacia and finally cystic cavity formation (porencephaly). Resolution of the inflammatory process and phagocytosis occurred before birth in both of these cases leaving no signs of inflammation. By the time animals were affected in the third trimester, only small numbers of glioblasts are present and only microscopic subependymal glial nodules are seen without gross malformations.

Although the fetus responded with an inflammatory glial reaction, neutralizing antibodies to the bluetongue virus were not seen until the beginning of the third trimester. The infections that produced hydranencephaly and porencephalic cysts left no evidence of their infectious nature. The importance of the susceptibility of a specific cell population of immature cells was shown with these bluetongue virus experiments since only cells in the subependymal germinal matrix were affected. Not all of the fetuses that were inoculated become infected. Infections at different stages of gestation produced different defects. The selective vulnerability of the telencephalic germinal matrix was not dependent upon the fact that this area was immature or that mitotic activity was occurring there since mitotic activity and immaturity are present in other cell populations at this time.[53]

Infection of fetal cats with feline ataxia virus has been shown to produce cerebellar hypoplasia of kittens.[92, 93] Clinically, this is manifested by ataxia. Other developing cell populations in the nervous system were not affected. This points out the specificity of viruses for certain cell populations within the developing nervous system.

Viruses that induced aqueductal stenosis and secondary hydrocephalus resembling agenesis of the aqueduct of Sylvius were first described after mumps virus infection in hamsters in 1967.[94] The growth of the mumps virus was limited to the ependymal cells and occasionally involved meningeal cells. After infection, the virus could not be recovered. No detectable antigen was found and no inflammatory response was present in the brain of these hydrocephalic hamsters at birth. If they were sacrificed at various stages of embryogenesis, it was seen that, following inoculation, a clinically apparent infection of the ependymal calls occurred that was associated with a pronounced perivascular inflammatory response. The inflammation resolved, but the loss of ependymal cells and subsequent overgrowth of glial elements produced stenosis (occlusion) of the aqueduct of Sylvius.[95] In this way the aqueductal stenosis with subsequent development of hydrocephalus was produced. At the time of birth there was an absence of inflammatory cells in these animals. The presence of aqueductal stenosis secondary to forking of the aqueduct with glial proliferation and ependymal rosette formation characterizes human and experimental aqueductal stenosis and subsequent hydrocephalus. Although there are some forms of aqueductal stenosis that are genetically determined,[96] in most cases, no genetic background for the hydrocephalus secondary to aqueductal stenosis can be found. The situation produced in the animal experiments is analogous to that seen in humans.[95]

These experiments point out the potential of viral infections to cause malformations of the brain in different stages of neuroembryogenesis. Each of the malformations described in these studies have their counterpart in man. These studies demonstrate that teratogens, specifically viruses, have the potential to cause central nervous system developmental anomalies that are seen in man. Proof of the viral etiology of these developmental defects in man is lacking because pathological signs of infection are absent at the time of birth when the disease is clinically manifested.

The most significant development of the central nervous system occurs during early gestation (prior to twenty-four weeks). The clinician should be aware of central nervous system manifestations secondary to genetic and/or chromosomal factors because subsequent pregnancies from the same parents may be affected. Many of the nongenetically or nonchromosomal determined abnormalities have been shown to be secondary to teratogens, specifically viruses.

Chapter 4

SPECIAL PROBLEMS OF THE NEONATAL NERVOUS SYSTEM AND THEIR RELATIONSHIP TO THE PRODUCTION OF DEVELOPMENTAL DISABILITIES

FACTORS ETIOLOGIC in producing brain damage, which subsequently may result in developmental disability, often occur in the neonatal period. Any factor that interferes with brain homeostasis may result in brain damage. The process may be primary such as meningoencephalitis or secondary to a peripheral one such as hypoxia.[97] Direct factors that may be associated with brain damage in the neonate include infection and trauma.[98, 99] Infections may rarely take the form of abscess of the brain which is an infection localized to one or more areas of the brain and by its nature will produce destruction of nervous system tissue.[100] More often, the infection takes the form of meningitis or properly stated, meningoencephalitis. Meningoencephalitis may result from viral, bacterial, protozoan, or fungal type infections.[101] In the neonate, it is rarely simply an infection of the meninges (the covering of the brain), but an infection involving the brain substance itself. Often in this process there is a vasculitis that may lead to thrombosis of the small blood vessels producing a series of small areas of infarction or stroke. The inflammation often spreads to the areas around the blood vessels in the brain causing inflammation and edema or swelling within these areas of the brain. The type of processes that occur depend upon the type of organism causing the meningoencephalitis, the severity of the infection, and the rapidity with which therapy is initiated.[101]

Fortunately, with the refinements in obstetrical techniques, the incidence of central nervous system trauma secondary to the birth process has been on the decline.[98,102] Trauma still may be etiologic in producing damage to the neonate's nervous system.

60

Trauma produces its damage by causing actual contusion of the brain with bleeding and swelling in these areas. At times, if the trauma is severe there may be frank hemorrhage into the brain substance itself. Occasionally with trauma, there is the production of subdural hematoma. The subdural hematoma by definition is a blood collection that lies in the cranium beneath the dura (one of the coverings of the brain). In and of itself, a subdural hematoma does not involve the brain tissue. However, the traumatic process which leads to the production of the subdural hematoma usually produces some contusion or bruising of the brain. This may occur in the area under the subdural or in an area opposite the primary site of trauma on the basis of the coup contre coup phenomenon.[103] Fortunately, because of the expansile capacity of the neonatal skull, neurosurgical intervention is rarely needed for treatment of the neonatal subdural hematoma.[104] The natural history of the hematoma is to resolve with time. Because the newborn's cranium can expand if the process is not acute, the subdural itself will not produce further brain damage if left to resolve on its own.

Secondary factors that may be etiologic in producing brain damage would include hormonal, nutritional, toxic, metabolic, and hypoxic factors.[105, 106, 107] Any factor that will interfere with the brain's oxygenation, removal of toxic metabolites or the loss of glucose (which is the natural energy substrate of the brain) will have the potential for producing brain damage. The hormonal factor that is well known as an etiologic factor in producing developmental disabilities is a lack of thyroid hormone. When there is a paucity or absence of thyroid hormone in the fetus or neonate, there is the potential for brain damage.[69, 70] Brain damage will occur if replacement hormone therapy is not instituted.[108] In this particular instance, the brain appears to be normally formed yet the cells do not have the proper interconnections that allow for normal intellectual function.

Nutritional factors as an etiology of brain damage and subsequent developmental disabilities have really been overrated.[71] The central nervous system has a definite precedence over other parts of the body when there is a lack of sufficient nutrition.

However, in very severe protein or general malnutrition, central nervous system damage may occur.[109]

Any metabolite that interferes with normal brain homeostasis may result in the production of nerve cell damage.[105] Bilirubin is a body metabolite known to produce brain cell damage in the newborn. This leads to a condition known as kernicterus.[110] In the newborn period, particularly in the premature, the blood brain barrier has not sufficiently matured so that unconjugated bilirubin may penetrate through the blood brain barrier and into the nervous system cells where it acts as a toxin. There are certain areas of the brain that are more susceptible to the bilirubin toxin. These areas include the basal ganglia, which are parts of the brain that exert an effect on the facility of muscle movement. It is the immaturity of the blood brain barrier that causes the difficulty. A high serum bilirubin in an older infant or child does not produce nerve cell damage.[111] There are many other metabolic products that can cause sufficient disruption in nervous cell metabolism to produce nerve cell damage and/or death, e.g. ammonia and other byproducts of protein metabolism.

Nerve cells are in a constant state of electrolyte balance. This balance is mediated by the neuronal cell membrane, which is electrically charged. When there is a significant electrolyte or pH imbalance there may be disturbance of cellular homeostasis.[105] Fortunately, in only severe instances does this lead to nerve cell damage or death. Electrolyte imbalances may cause instability of the nerve cell membrane and subsequently result in the production of seizures. Seizures may occur at the time of imbalance, during the dynamic period of imbalance correction, or after the imbalance has been corrected if the cell membrane has been permanently altered.

The metabolite that the brain requires for normal cellular activity is glucose.[112] Processes that deprive the brain of glucose may subsequently disrupt the cells so that they die or become impaired. Unfortunately, the brain has only limited other mechanisms for energy metabolism to temporarily alleviate the need for glucose. Different cell populations within the brain are differentially sensitive to a decrease in glucose or oxygen.

A most critical factor for brain cell function is oxygen.[112] It is with sufficient oxygenation that metabolic reactions within these cells can take place and the toxic by-products eliminated. Any process that will diminish or eliminate the brain's ability to receive oxygen may result in the production of neuronal damage. Processes such as respiratory distress syndrome (hyaline membrane disease) may prevent normal oxygenation of the blood. In this condition, there is immaturity of the lungs. Often this condition is seen in premature infants.[113] Processes that produce hypotension or hypoprofusion of the brain may also lead to decreased oxygen in the nervous system.[114, 115]

Generally, when neurotoxic processes occur, they involve the entire central nervous system.[105, 112] It is distinctly unusual for only specific focal areas to be involved in such a process.[116] The one exception would be the occurrence of emboli to the blood vessels in the brain which would produce focal discrete areas of infarction or brain cell death. Embolic processes are unusual in the newborn.[117] Usually, the neurotoxic process is diffuse and produces a diffuse encephalopathy. However, the insult may induce more damage in some areas than in others. At times, this relates to the nature of the insult, as in hyperbilirubinemia where the basal ganglia are affected with a greater propensity than other portions of the nervous system.

Diffuse neurotoxic agents may select some areas based on the peculiar vascular anatomy of each individual's nervous system[118] and the selective vulnerability of certain cell populations.[119] Neurotoxic insults in the newborn producing brain damage are *not* analogous to the situation in an adult where there is a stroke and one particular area of the brain is destroyed and other areas are totally unaffected. It is this concept of the diffuseness of neonatal nervous system insults that makes it unlikely that other areas of the nervous system can develop, renew function, and cause the individual to assume normal function. This does not occur because these injuries are diffuse, although some areas are affected with greater severity. To support this concept one can look to situations where individuals with normal nervous systems have had to receive hemispherectomies prior to the age of three years.[120] In these instances, there is relatively little if any demonstrable loss of psychomotor function. This is taken in direct contrast to the child who has experienced some diffuse insult picking out some areas more than others, who is not able to achieve normal psychomotor development and function.

Injury to cells of the nervous system may result in producing cell death, cell damage, a defect in dendritic arborization, and/or a defect in normal myelination.[101, 121, 122] If there is cellular death, this produces a loss of neurons and loss of their nerve cell processes and, therefore, a diminution of the amount of white and gray matter that is seen. This may result in the production of a developmental delay provided the entire cell population has not been destroyed. The severity of the delay would correlate with the severity of the injury. The result of this type of insult often can be seen on special x-ray studies such as the CAT (computerized axial tomographic) scan where one would see an increase in the ventricular system (the hollow spaces inside the brain) (Figure 19) and an increase in the width and depth of the sulci of the cortex.[123] In these instances, the areas of cell and white matter loss are filled in with cerebrospinal fluid that naturally bathes the interior and exterior portions of the brain. This produces a condition known as hydrocephalus ex vacuo. In very severe injuries, there is a loss of neuronal cells and a lack or decrease of further brain development resulting in the production of microcephaly. Unfortunately, there is no treatment for this process.

If the neuronal cells are damaged, there may be an alteration in the cells' excitability or an alteration in the cells' function. The manifestations vary according to areas damaged and the severity of the injury. The alteration in cytofunction in hyperbilirubinemia where the basal ganglia are damaged produces a movement disorder. The damage of other neuronal cells may result in an altered threshold of excitability, which may subsequently lead to a lowered threshold for seizure production.[124]

The means by which we convey information from cell to cell within our nervous system is by interconnections mediated by the dendritic tree. Dendrites are processes that pick up information from other cells in the nervous system. It is in this manner that all of our neurons are interconnected. The process of neuronal cell interconnection begins before birth and continues throughout life.[127] There have been a number of experiments in animals and observations in pathological states in humans showing that neurotoxic processes may lead to a delay in the proliferation of the cellular dendrites and defective arborization of the dendritic tree and intercellular hook-up.[122, 125, 126] The manifestation of the defect is a delay in the acquisition of developmental skills. The ultimate level of performance of these skills is diminished. This is analogous to what is seen in individuals who have developmental disabilities where they acquire skills at a slower rate and usually do not achieve as sophisticated ultimate levels of performance as a normal individual.

Neurotoxic events may lead to delay in the laying down of myelin in the central nervous system, but myelination does occur.[127] The total decrease in myelin often reflects the decrease in neuronal cell populations and, therefore, the number of myelinated cell processes. The lack of myelin formation may be a reflection of the lack of neuronal cells and myelinated cell processes. Diminution in myelin may be overrated as an etiological factor in producing developmental disabilities and may be the secondary event. Certainly, there are conditions where there is a defect in myelination and a regression in development.[128, 129] However, in these conditions, there is also production of toxic metabolites that interfere with cell function (Appendix A and B).

Unfortunately, after the newborn infant has suffered a neurotoxic insult, there often is little in the way of physical signs of damage. The signs of damage become apparent as the infant matures into childhood. The nervous system of the newborn infant is indeed very primitive, and, to point this out most dramatically, one could look at the hydranencephalic infant (an infant who lacks most if not all of the cerebral cortex).[130] There is little functional difference between the normal newborn and hydranencephalic infant except the normal newborn is capable of fixing and following on objects where the hydranencephalic is not.

Although infants may have experienced one or more of these

neurotoxic insults, the result may not necessarily be the production of brain damage. There are other critical factors involved such as the age of onset of treatment, e.g. thyroid hormone for cretinism, and the gestational age, e.g. infant exposed to hyperbilirubinemia. The length of time the neonate is exposed to an insult, the severity of the insult, and the exposure to multiple insults will influence the risk of brain damage and subsequent developmental disabilities.

Neonatal seizures and neonatal intracranial hemorrhage are two processes that occur with great frequency and are often associated with brain damage and subsequent developmental disability. It is because of these factors that the remainder of the chapter will be devoted to these two phenomena.

Neonatal Intraventricular Hemorrhage

Initially, it was assumed that intraventricular hemorrhage was the result of birth trauma or coagulation deficits. However, further investigations revealed that this is not the case, that intraventricular hemorrhage is more common in premature infants and indeed has been inversely correlated with gestational age. It has also been directly correlated with the occurrence of hyaline membrane disease.[131]

The association with prematurity and the location of the hemorrhages has caused researchers to look into the anatomy of the premature infant.[131-136] They have found that the hemorrhages originate in the subependymal germinal matrix (Chapter 3). This is the area that is close to the ventricles where neuronal cells (until twenty-four weeks of gestation) and glial cells (until approximately four weeks postnatally) are made. The blood vessels in this area, particularly the venules, have a very characteristic anatomy. The venules are very thin-walled structures with poor muscular coats. They are patulous and friable. It is from the venules in this ependymal germinal matrix that the intraventricular hemorrhage originates. The subependymal germinal matrix resolves as the fetus matures and, by four weeks postnatal life, the subependymal germinal matrix has completely resolved. This correlates with the relationship of the frequency of intraventricular hemorrhage at lower gestational ages.

The specific factors that lead to the production of the hemorrhage have not been clearly elucidated. However, factors that have been incriminated include hypoxia, hypotension, and hypertension. Perhaps, it is one of the factors or a combination of all three that cause the rupture of the venules in the subependymal germinal matrix. The premature infant is vulnerable to neurotoxic insults of a general nature, but he is prone to hemorrhage, which may cause focal destruction of brain tissue.

In addition, the presence of blood in the ventricles and in the spinal fluid may lead to blockage in the normal spinal fluid flow.[137] Spinal fluid is made in the human at the rate of 0.36 ml per minute and is reabsorbed at the same rate. The spinal fluid is made in specialized structures within the ventricle called the choroid plexus. The fluid then circulates through the ventricular system (Figure 19) through specific passages in the brain

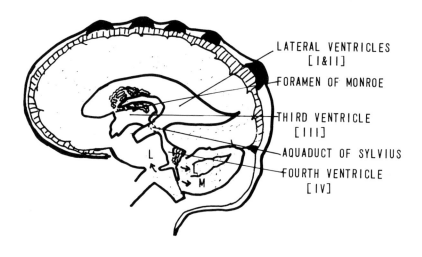

LATERAL VENTRICLES [I&II]

FORAMEN OF MONROE

THIRD VENTRICLE [III]

AQUADUCT OF SYLVIUS

FOURTH VENTRICLE [IV]

Chorioid Plexus

Pacchionian Granules

FORAMINA OF MAGENDIE [M] AND LUSCHKA [L]

Figure 19. Formation, circulation, and reabsorption of cerebrospinal fluid. Spinal fluid is made by the choroid plexus in the ventricular system, flows through a series of channels and exits through the foramina of Magendie and Luschka to circulate in the subarachnoid space and be reabsorbed at the Pacchionian granules.

substance to reach the subarachnoid space (space under the outside covering of the brain) and it is in specialized structures (pacchionian granules) within the lumbo-subarachnoid space that the spinal fluid is reabsorbed.[138] The presence of foreign materials such as blood or pus may lead to a disruption in the normal system of spinal fluid flow, produce inflammatory reactions, and secondarily produce a condition of hydrocephalus.[137, 139]

In hydrocephalus, normal passage of spinal fluid is blocked (noncommunicating hydrocephalus) or normal reabsorption of the spinal fluid cannot occur (communicating hydrocephalus).[140] This results in a condition of excessive fluid accumulation and increased pressure within the cranium and the development of a large head in individuals who have the capacity to expand their cranium. In some newborns, the presence of blood may only temporarily disrupt the normal cerebrospinal fluid dynamics and the process spontaneously resolves.[141] However, in most instances, this is permanent and neurosurgical intervention with a shunting procedure (placing a plastic tube in the hollow space of the brain to another body cavity) must be undertaken.

It was felt that the presence of intraventricular hemorrhage was a severe life-threatening situation with a 44 percent mortality.[142] However, the frequent use of the computerized axial tomographic brain scan in newborns has shown that many more infants experience intraventricular hemorrhage than previously noted since only the most severely affected infants were initially studied.[143] In actuality, the mortality from intraventricular hemorrhage is considerably less. However, it is a factor that may be associated with the production of developmental disabilities. Most infants who experience intracranial intraventricular hemorrhage experience the hemorrhage between fifteen and forty-eight hours of age (60%). Only 16 percent of individuals who experience intraventricular hemorrhage will have their hemorrhage before twenty-four hours of age. The single most commonly associated symptom with the intraventricular bleed is the onset of seizures. Other factors that have been associated with intracranial hemorrhage include a sudden drop in hematocrit, bradycardia, apnea, and a tense fontanelle.[142] The only treatment for intraventricular hemorrhage is symptomatic.

Neonatal Seizures

Seizures occur frequently in the neonatal period (birth to twenty-eight days). They occur in approximately 1.2 percent of live born infants. The seizures of the neonate bear certain differences from seizures seen in older infants, children, or adults.[144-150] Their peripheral manifestations differ, their etiologies differ, their electroencephalographic correlations differ, their prognosis differs and even their treatment is somewhat unique. Unlike seizures in the older infant or child, neonatal seizures in and of themselves do not often constitute a threat to basic body function. Many neonates who experience seizures are capable of feeding and carrying out normal infant activities, although they may be intermittently experiencing a seizure activity. It is for this reason that neonatal seizures may often go unrecognized until they become severe and resemble the seizures seen in the more mature nervous system.

The types of neonatal seizures include subtle, focal clonic, multifocal clonic, tonic, myclonic, and jittery. The subtle type of neonatal seizure is the most common form, yet this form of seizure is most often overlooked because its manifestations are often misinterpreted as random baby activity. These seizures consist of any subtle nonvoluntary motor activity, such as tonic horizontal deviations of the eyes with or without nystagmoid jerks, oral buccal movements much like sucking, drooling, masticatory movements of the mouth, repetitive fluttering of the eyelids, stiffening of the limbs for seconds, abnormal limb movements, slight tremors of the limbs, apnea, bradycardia, etc. Apnea and bradycardia are not uncommon manifestations of neonatal seizures. Many newborns who have seizures may be incorrectly labeled as benign apnea of prematurity or as near-miss sudden infant death.

Focal clonic seizures are a frequently observed seizure pattern. They usually are localized, occurring about the face or one limb and consist of jerky or clonic (shaking) movements in these structures. They spread slowly and intermittently to other parts of the body. These often wax and wane and, like the subtle seizure, do not cause unconsciousness and do not interfere with other body functions such as feeding. It is important to emphasize that focal seizures in the neonate are commonly manifestations of diffuse cerebral insult; they lack the specificity of focal disease that one associates with focal seizures in the older child or adult.

Multifocal clonic seizures (also known as fragmentary or migratory) are characterized by shifting clonic movements migrating rapidly from one part of the body to another in a non-Jacksonian fashion (no particular anatomical pattern). They may occur rapidly and culminate in a generalized seizure. These seizures do interfere with body functions and usually cause the child to be brought to medical attention.

The tonic seizure is a seizure of stiffening; these may be focal or generalized. When they are generalized, they may appear as peculiar neurological posturings such as decerebrate, decorticate or opistotonic. If they are focal, they consist simply of stiffening of one limb or pairs of limbs on one side of the body. When these are generalized, they usually come to medical attention.

Myoclonic jerks are usually rather synchronous movements of large muscle groups or single jerks of a limb and/or pairs of limbs and/or all four limbs. The episode lasts but for a second and may resemble the startle response of the normal newborn. These may occur in a migratory fragmentary state or simply as synchronous jerking of one extremity.

Jitteriness is a symptom that may reflect a metabolic disturbance or may reflect withdrawal of neurotrophic medications. However, jitteriness may be the manifestations of neonatal seizures. Although this is hard to discern from jitteriness of other etiologies, jitteriness of seizures is often associated with abnormal extraocular movements and other subtle seizure phenomena.

Unfortunately, many neonatal seizures, particularly jitteriness, are stimulus sensitive and also stimulus quiescent. A person may stimulate seizures by activating the baby or may quiet the seizures by stimulating the baby. In addition to the motor manifestations of the neonatal seizures, autonomic nervous system dysfunction may be produced. The infant with seizures may appear hyperemic, may have a drop in blood pressure or a rise in blood pressure, a drop in pulse, a rise in pulse, a peculiarity of breathing pattern, a cessation of breathing or rapid breathing, a rise in temperature or a lowering in temperature. In essence, any functions of the autonomic nervous system may be dysfunctional during, before or after an infant has experienced a seizure. Since it is difficult to distinguish seizure activity from random baby activity (particularly in the forms of subtle neonatal seizures), it is important for the physician, nurse or parent to observe the infant and to compare his activity with normal newborn activity. It is only by making this comparison that a prompt diagnosis of seizure can be made in the early stages.

Neonatal seizures may be a reflection of nervous system irritability or may be a reflection of nervous system damage with a lowered threshold to spontaneous firing. Any of the factors mentioned earlier in this chapter which are neurotoxic may lead to the production of seizures. Electrolyte disturbances such as hypocalcemia, hypernatremia, hyponatremia, hypomagnesiumemia, intracranial hemorrhage, birth trauma, infection and hypoglycemia, etc., all may lead to seizures. In addition, infants who have congenital cerebral malformations are likely to have seizures at any point in life and may have seizures in the newborn period. Perinatal hypoxia is a commonly experienced factor in the newborn period and it may be etiologic in producing seizures.

The potential for the development of seizures later during life depends on the etiology of the neonatal seizures.[146] For example, a simple hypocalcemic seizure in the newborn period carries a rather good prognosis for not having seizures later in life as well as not having serious brain damage and subsequent developmental disabilities. However, the prognosis with other factors is not quite as optimistic. The child with congenital cerebral malformation would have a high risk of having seizures later in life, as well as having brain damage and developmental disability. In every case of neonatal seizures, the prognosis is variable depending upon the factors that produced the seizure in the individual. However, in general, if one has experienced an insult to the degree that seizure activity has occurred, there is a chance of having permanent brain damage and subsequent developmental disability later in life. This has been reflected in studies on cerebral palsy individuals where the coincidence of neonatal seizures was associated with a poorer prognosis.

In treating neonatal seizures, one must not only use anticonvulsants promptly but also look for any metabolic disturbance that may have been etiologic in producing the seizure because, should a metabolic disturbance be present, it must be corrected promptly.

In the older child and in the adult, seizures in and of themselves are not taken to be etiologic in producing brain damage.[151] In these individuals, they are at risk from damage with seizures because of the occasionally associated hypoxia, hypoglycemia, hypothermia, and hypoprofusion that may accompany the seizure as a manifestation of autonomic nervous system instability.[23] However, in the neonate, there is some evidence that neonatal seizures in and of themselves may be etiologic in producing brain damage.[152, 153] It is for this reason that it is important to promptly recognize and treat neonatal seizures.

Chapter 5

THE HEAD: MACROCEPHALY, MICROCEPHALY, AND ABERRANT CONFIGURATIONS

THE SIZE AND CONFIGURATION of an individual's head is dependent upon genetic factors, the timing of the closure of the cranial sutures and fontanelles, environmental factors, and intercranial processes. In many children with developmental disabilities, aberrations of cranial configuration and size reflect intercranial processes.[154] The normal growth of the skull depends on normal brain growth and normal timetable of closure of fontanelles and skull sutures. Normally the posterior fontanelle closes at six to eight weeks and the anterior fontanelle at sixteen to eighteen months.[43]

Judgements concerning cranial configurations are made by inspection and by head circumference measurements. Head circumference measurements are compared with normal values based upon age and sex.[42] In an individual whose cranial configuration is abnormal, serial head measurements can be made by special techniques on skull x-ray and comparisons made with norms for age and sex.[155] In premature newborns, head circumference measurements can be compared with normal for gestational age and sex.[156] In prematures who have suffered perinatal illnesses, comparison can be made concerning their rate of change in head growth.[157, 158] In these prematures, it is the rate of change of head growth that is significant, since premature infants who have been seriously ill may have an initial slow period of head growth followed by a period of rapid catch-up growth. It is important to differentiate catch-up growth from early hydrocephalus. The recent refinement of computerized axial tomographic (CAT) scanning of the head has enabled clinicians to determine if intercranial pathology exists without using invasive procedures.[123, 159]

73

When confronted with an infant or child whose head circumference measurement is abnormal for age and sex it is important to observe the child for any stigmata of associative conditions[72, 160, 161] and to correlate the percentile rank for head size with the percentile rank for the child's height and weight. The significance of the child whose head circumference is at the third percentile but whose body height and weight are at the ninety-eighth percentile is different than a child whose head circumference is at the third percentile and whose height and weight are also at the third percentile. In the former case, one would be more concerned that the patient is developing microcephaly than one would be in the latter case. In most instances the judgement concerning an increase or decrease in head size is best made by serial determinations of head circumference over a period of time to determine the child's rate of change in head size. For example, if one were to have a head circumference at the tenth percentile which remained at the tenth percentile over a series of months one would be less concerned than if one had a child whose head circumference is at the tenth percentile but had been at the seventy-fifth and then at the twenty-fifth percentiles in the past.

Microcephaly can be defined as a head circumference that is below two standard deviations for normal (below the second percentile) and macrocephaly can be defined as a head circumference two standard deviations above normal (above the ninety-eighth percentile) for age and sex. The problems of macrocephaly, microcephaly, and aberrant skull configurations will be considered separately.

Macrocephaly

Macrocephaly can be defined as a head circumference greater than two standard deviations above normal for age and sex. In assessing the patient with macrocephaly it is important to perform a good general physical examination and a thorough neurological examination (Chapter 2) since the differential diagnosis of this condition is wide (see Table V). As part of a good neurological examination, transillumination of the skull can yield important information, provided the infant or young child

Table V

DIFFERENTIAL DIAGNOSIS OF MACROCEPHALY

I. Hydrocephalus.
   A. Congenital anomalies.
      1. Anomalies of the ventricular flow system.
         a. Atresia of aqueduct of Sylvius.
         b. Atresia of foramina of Luschka and Magendie.
      2. Anomalies with associated hydrocephalus.
         a. Arnold-Chiari malformation.
         b. Meningomyelocele.
         c. Encephalocele.
         d. Porencephalic cysts.
         e. Platybasia.
         f. Klippel-Feil deformity.
   B. Neoplasia.
      1. Growth and blockage of foramina, e.g. colloid cyst of third ventricle.
      2. Secondary effect of intracranial neoplasms without blockage of ventricular system.
      3. Choroid plexus tumors (with increased production of cerebrospinal fluid).
   C. Inflammation.
      1. Secondary to hemorrhage.
         a. Subependymal germinal matrix or choroid plexus hemorrhage in the neonate.
         b. Hemorrhage secondary to trauma.
         c. Hemorrhage secondary to rupture of vascular lesions, e.g. aneurysms, arteriovenous malformation.
      2. Secondary to infection.
         a. Brain abscess.
         b. Meningoencephalitis.
         c. Intrauterinely acquired infections.
      3. Secondary to noninfectious meningeal irritation.
         a. Leukemia.
         b. Metastatic neoplasms.
   D. Arachnoid cysts with blockage of ventricular flow.
   E. Vascular.
      1. Vein of Galen malformation.
      2. Thrombosis of venous sinuses.
   F. Toxin, e.g. lead.
II. Hydranencephaly.
III. Arachnoidal cysts.
IV. Subdural collections.
   A. Hematoma.
   B. Effusion.
   C. Empyema.
V. Scalp and bony collections.
   A. Osteogenesis imperfecta.
   B. Cephalohematomas or caput succedaneum in newborns.
   C. Local fluid collections, e.g. edema, blood, I.V. fluids.
VI. Metabolic disorders.
   A. Mucopolysaccharidosis.
   B. Storage and degenerative diseases, e.g. GM_2, GM_1, Alexander's, Krabbe's, Canavan's, etc.
   C. Dwarfism syndromes, e.g. achondroplasia.

Table V — *Continued*

D. Endocrine disorders, e.g. cerebral gigantism.
F. Aminoacidopathies, e.g. MSU.
VII. Pseudotumor cerebri.
    A. Hyper- or hypovitaminosis A.
    B. Tetracycline.
    C. Steroids.
    D. Hypoparathyroidism.
VIII. Neurocutaneous syndromes.
    A. Tuberosclerosis.
    B. Sturge-Weber syndrome.
    C. Neurofibromatosis.
  IX. Megencephaly.
    A. Benign familial.
    B. Symptomatic.

has little hair over the scalp.[44] Sometimes it may be necessary to measure the cranial size of the parents and other family members if one is considering a diagnosis of familial macrocephaly.[162]

Hydrocephalus

Hydrocephalus is the most frequent cause of macrocephaly. Hydrocephalus is a condition where there is an excessive accumulation of cerebrospinal fluid under pressure within the ventricular system or lumbosubarachnoid space. Hydrocephalus may be of two types. It may be communicating where there is no obstruction within the ventricular system of the brain (hollow spaces within the brain) or noncommunicating where there is an obstruction of the ventricular system within the confines of the brain (Figure 19).[163]

Congenital anomalies may be etiologic in producing hydrocephalus or may be associated with hydrocephalus. Anomalies of the ventricular flow system would produce hydrocephalus directly. The most common abnormality of ventricular flow is *atresia of the aqueduct of Sylvius*.[164] This blocks the ventricular fluid flow system between the third and fourth ventricles causing dilatation of the lateral ventricles and the third ventricle. Infants may be born with complete atresia of the aqueduct of Sylvius or may develop full occlusion of the aqueduct over the first few days or weeks of life. There is a genetic sex-linked recessive form of hydrocephalus secondary to atresia of the aqueduct of Sylvius.[96] Another anomaly that will produce a noncommunicating hydrocephalus is atresia of the foramen of Luschka and Magendie.[165] When this is associated with hypoplasia of the cerebellum and large cystic dilatation of the fourth ventricle as well as with hydrocephalus, it is called a *Dandy-Walker anomaly.*

Certain other congenital anomalies of the brain and bony coverings of the brain are associated with hydrocephalus. The most common of these is the *Arnold-Chiari malformation* where there is the displacement of posterior fossa contents (the medulla and/or cerebellum) into the cervical portion of the spinal cord on the basis of a maldevelopment of the cervical flexure during embryogenesis (Chapter 3).[166] The Arnold-Chiari malformation is associated with aqueductal stenosis. *Meningomyeloceles* and *spina bifidas* are also associated with hydrocephalus and with the Arnold-Chiari malformation.[167-169] *Encephaloceles* and *meningoencephaloceles* are also developmental defects in neuroembryogenesis which may be associated with hydrocephalus of either the communicating or the noncommunicating type.[168] *Porencephalic cysts* (Chapter 3) may be associated with communicating hydrocephalus.[170] *Platybasia* is a developmental anomaly that results from the upper displacement of the superior portion of the cervical spine into the posterior fossa causing an elevation of the floor of the posterior fossa and a reduction in its capacity. As a result, there is a compression of the cerebellum and a downward displacement of some cerebellar tissue. The Arnold-Chiari malformation may be associated with this. Atlantoaxial fusions may occur, and meningobulbia may be seen as well.[171]

The *Klippel-Feil deformity* is also associated with hydrocephalus. This is a failure of the normal segmentation of cervical vertebrae so that there are fewer cervical vertebrae. Those present may be malformed. This condition may be associated with spina bifidas of the cervical area. The afflicted person usually has a very short neck. Meningoceles or meningomyeloceles of the cervical area are seen with this deformity and Sprengel's deformity is also associated with this condition.[172] Sprengel's deformity is a congenital elevation of the scapula (shoulder blade).[173]

Neoplasms may be associated with hydrocephalus in several ways. Their growth may produce blockage in the ventricular system and cause a noncommunicating hydrocephalus. This may be seen with colloid cysts of the third ventricle. Neoplasms may also cause communicating hydrocephalus because of their secondary effect in the intracranial cavity producing swelling and edema of the brain.[174] A specialized form of tumor of the choroid plexus may also be etiologic in producing hydrocephalus. Choroid plexus tumors cause hydrocephalus by producing an amount of cerebrospinal fluid that exceeds the capacity of the individual's spinal flow system to reabsorb spinal fluid (Figure 19).[175]

Inflammatory processes may also lead to hydrocephalus.[137, 139] These can be secondary to hemorrhage, infection, or noninfectious meningeal irritants. A *hemorrhage* produces hydrocephalus by either causing a direct blockage of ventricular fluid flow or by causing a reaction in the lumbosubarachnoid space so that the cerebrospinal fluid cannot be reabsorbed at its normal rate. A frequent cause of hemorrhage leading to hydrocephalus in the neonate is a hemorrhage from the subependymal germinal matrix (Chapter 4) or hemorrhage from the choroid plexus.[142] Hemorrhage secondary to trauma, either trauma during birth or trauma at any point in life, may also lead to blockage of CSF reabsorption or flow. Hemorrhage may be secondary to rupture of vascular lesions such as aneurysms or arteriovenous malformations.[174]

Infections may produce alterations in cerebrospinal fluid dynamics so as to cause hydrocephalus. *Brain abscesses* may cause hydrocephalus by their growth and blockage of ventricular foramine or by causing a mass effect within the cranium, producing edema and increased cerebrospinal fluid pressure.[174] Infection may likewise cause aberrations in CSF flow dynamics, either by creating a severe ventriculitis or by a mechanical blockage of spinal fluid flow through the ventricular system or by causing an inflammatory reaction about the pacchionian granules (Figure 19) and thereby preventing reabsorption of cerebrospinal fluid at the normal rate.[139] *Intrauterine acquired infections* may lead to the production of hydrocephalus by the blockage of ventricular flow or by prevention of reabsorption of cerebrospinal fluid.[176] Infectious processes that are associated with this phenomena are toxoplasmosis and cytomegalic virus inclusion disease. There are processes causing *meningeal irritation* of a noninfectious or nonhemorrhagic nature such as *leukemia* and *metastatic neoplasms*.[177] These processes may lead to poor reabsorption of cerebrospinal fluid through the pacchionian granules (Figure 19).

Arachnoid cysts of a developmental nature may cause blockage of the ventricular flow system and thereby produce hydrocephalus.[174] *Vascular aberrations* may also be responsible for producing hydrocephalus.[178-180] Anomalies of the vein of Galen may, because of their size and location, put pressure on the ventricular flow system causing noncommunicating hydrocephalus. *Thrombosis* of venous sinuses may occur, e.g. with severe electrolyte imbalance and dehydration, and may produce a defect in venous drainage from the cranium causing congestion in the brain and poor reabsorptive capacity of the pacchionian granules for cerebrospinal fluid.

Other Causes of Macrocephaly

Hydranencephaly is a developmental anomaly of the brain (Chapter 3), which may be associated with macrocephaly. In hydranencephaly, there is a lack of development of the cerebral hemispheres (except possibly for occipital and inferior temporal lobes) and there may be a large collection of fluid expanding in the cranium producing macrocephaly. These individuals have a normal skull and normal meninges. The transillumination pattern in hydranencephaly is very characteristic with pronounced transilumination of the entire skull and light being transmitted through the pupils. This is known as the jack-o-lantern sign.[44]

Arachnoid cysts may enlarge and secondarily produce enlargement of the skull. Oftentimes growing arachnoid cysts will produce focal cranial enlargement.

Subdural collections may be responsible for enlargement of the skull. Subdural hematomas may occur after trauma. If the cranial sutures are not fused they may produce enlargement of the skull.[104] Acute subdural hematomas may require immediate surgical intervention, but subacute and chronic forms will often resolve without therapeutic intervention provided there is a freely expansible cranium.[104, 174, 181] Subdural effusions may occur secondary to resolution of subdural hematomas, in which case they may become subdural hygromas. Subdural effusions may occur secondary to infectious processes, e.g. Hemophilus influenza and pneumococcal meningitis. Subdural empyemas may also cause enlargement of the skull. Subdural empyemas by definition are collections of pus in the subdural space. These infections may be secondary to meningoencephalitis or trauma.

Any process that will cause a *thickening of the scalp or bone* of the skull will lead to macrocephaly. Conditions of the bones such as osteogenesis imperfecta[182] and severe anemia[183] (causing extramedullary hematopoiesis within the skull bones) may lead to enlargement of the cranium. In rare instances, bony tumors may also proliferate to such a degree that macrocephaly or abnormal configuration of the skull is produced.[174] In newborns, hematomas of the subperiosteal areas called cephalohematomas may also occur and cause a localized enlargement of the head. In newborns, fluid and blood collections may occur secondary to traumatic passage through the birth canal. These fluid blood collections are called caput succedaneum and resolve rather rapidly without intervention. In the newborn period, local fluid collections within the scalp from severe edema, from blood secondary to trauma, or from infiltration from intravenous feedings may lead to enlargement of the scalp and macrocephaly. However, these processes are rapidly reversible without therapeutic intervention.[184]

There are certain *metabolic conditions* that are associated with macrocephaly. Conditions such as mucopolysaccharidosis and other forms of storage and degenerative diseases may be responsible for macrocephaly (Appendix B). There are some syndromes of dwarfism in which there is a true macrocephaly. Forms of achondroplasia are often associated with macrocephaly and, in some instances, may be associated with true hydrocephalus as well.[185] Maple syrup urine disease, a form of aminoacidopathy (Appendix A) may be associated with macrocephaly. Cerebral gigantism, where the individual has developmental disabilities and macrosomatia, may be associated with macrocephaly.[186]

If *pseudotumorous cerebri* occurs in individuals whose sutures have not fused there may be macrocephaly.[187] Pseudotumorous cerebri is a diagnosis of exclusion in which there is increased cerebrospinal fluid pressure with small ventricles. Although the etiology of this condition is often unknown, it has been associated with obese adolescent females, hypovitaminosis A, ingestion of tetracycline, hypoparathyroidism and steroid medication.

Many of the *neurocutaneous syndromes* (Appendix C) are associated with a true macrocephaly. Tuberosclerosis, Sturge-Weber, and neurofibromatosis may be associated with true macrocephaly.

True macrocephaly does exist. There are some families where megencephaly is asymptomatic.[162] In these families, one or both parents will have head circumferences above the ninety-eighth percentile for age and not have any neurological handicap. Children who are given a diagnosis of benign familial megencephaly should have had all other causes of macrocephaly excluded. There is a symptomatic form of megencephaly where the children have large brains and developmental disabilities.[101, 188] This may be genetic, but the parents are asymptomatic with normal skulls. Individuals with true megencephaly have large heads with thickening of the cortex and the subcortical white matter. Their ventricles may also be slightly dilated and neuropathologically they may show neuronal heterotopias (Chapter 3). There is a significant increase in the frequency of males affected as compared to females leading to a question of a sex-linked genetic pattern. Approximately half of the individuals with true megencephaly will have seizure disorders. The hallmark of true megencephaly is a symmetrically enlarged head, developmental delays, seizures, and no evidence of other brain pathology.

Microcephaly

Microcephaly is defined as a head circumference below the second percentile for age and sex. Microcephaly can be secondary to constitutional factors or secondary to acquired neurotoxic insults. Microcephalic skulls tend to have premature synostosis of the sutures and premature closure of the fontanelles. This is a reflection of poor brain growth. In these instances, closure of the sutures are not etiologic in producing microcephaly, but the premature closure of the sutures are secondary to defective brain growth.[154] It is unnecessary to have suture stripping procedures in individuals with true microcephaly since this will not change their skull configuration nor alter their brain growth. In the evaluation of a child with suspected microcephaly, serial head circumference measurements over time are important.

Table VI
DIFFERENTIAL DIAGNOSIS OF MICROCEPHALY

I. Constitutional.
   A. Genetic.
      1. Benign familial.
      2. Symptomatic familial.
         a. Autosomal recessive.
         b. Cockayne's syndrome.
         c. X-linked recessive.
         d. Seckel's bird-headed dwarf.
      3. Associated with storage and degenerative diseases.
      4. Associated with aminoacidopathies.
   B. Chromosomal.
      1. Down's syndrome (Trisomy 21).
      2. Trisomy D (13-15).
      3. Trisomy E (17-18).
      4. Cri du chat.
      5. Ring chromosome 18.
      6. Chromosomal deletions or additions, e.g. 4p-.
   C. Associated with defined syndromes.
      1. Beckwith's syndrome.
      2. Rubinstein-Taybi syndrome.
      3. Smith-Lemli-Opitz syndrome.
      4. Cornelia de Lange's syndrome.
II. Acquired.
   A. Intrauterine.
      1. Infection.
      2. Radiation.
      3. Hypoxia.
      4. Toxic (alcohol).
      5. Hormonal (uncontrolled diabetes).
   B. Acquired perinatal.
      1. Hypoxia.
      2. Infection.
      3. Other.

With serial measurement one can determine the overall trend in skull and brain development. In general, individuals with acquired microcephaly will have initial head circumferences within the normal percentiles but as they advance in age their head circumference will cross percentile lines and rest below the third percentile for age and sex. The differential diagnosis of microcephaly is extensive (see Table VI).

Constitutional

Although hereditary forms of microcephaly are relatively uncommon, they do constitute approximately 6 percent of institutionalized patients with microcephaly.[189-191] Most forms of symptomatic genetic microcephaly conform to a recessive mode of inheritance. In genetic forms of microcephaly, the skull configuration often is different than individuals who have acquired microcephaly. In individuals with genetic forms of microcephaly, there is a tendency for a narrow head with a sloping forehead and a marked reduction in vertical diameter of the head. The face and the ears usually appear normal in size. The individual's mental capacity is usually moderately to severely delayed. The individuals often have a short stature. These individuals often have premature synostosis of their cranial sutures. Pathologically, their brains are small. The gyri are well formed but there may be a simplified convolutional pattern to the brain in a columnar arrangement of neurons. There is a genetic form of microcephaly that is sex-linked recessive in which there is lissencephaly (lack of gyri and sulci) of the cerebral cortex.[192] Clinically, these patients have profound developmental delay and do not acquire language. They are usually blind and bed-ridden throughout their lives. Individuals with other forms of genetic microcephaly usually have normal or almost normal motor milestones, but their speech and other developmental milestones are markedly delayed. Many individuals with genetic forms of microcephaly never develop functional language.

A form of familial microcephaly associated with intercranial calcification and autosomal and recessive in character is *Cockayne's syndrome*.[193, 194] Individuals with Cockayne's syndrome have dwarfism, a beaked nose, dermatitis in a butterfly distribution about their face, and seizure disorder. They appear normal at birth but have a progressive downhill course and may well represent a form of degenerative disease. Pathologically, their brains are small in size and there are calcium deposits in the cortex, basal ganglia, dentate nucleus, thalamus, and red nucleus. Microcephaly may be associated with some forms of *aminoacidopathies* (Appendix A). *Alper's disease* is a familial condition that is associated with microcephaly.[195] In this condition, there are also seizures and myoclonus, severe developmental disability, and a progressive degenerative course.

There is an uncommonly encountered pedigree where family members have small heads and no significant neurological findings.[196] This is an exceptionally rare entity, but a clue to this diagnosis would be a normal development in the child with a small head whose family members are normal neurologically and have small heads.

Chromosomal syndromes (Appendix C) are often associated with microcephaly. In addition to the microcephaly, other congenital anomalies are seen with these conditions.

Microcephaly is also seen with many *other forms of presumably genetic disorders.*[72, 160, 161] The *Cornelia de Lange's syndrome* is a condition where microcephaly, severe developmental delay, short stature, synophrys (midline fusion of the eyebrows) occurs. In addition there are other minor anomalies such as micrognathia, small beaked nose, carp-like mouths, increased length of the frenulum (distance between the nose and the upper lip), finger anomalies, and cardiac anomalies. The *Smith-Lemli-Opitz syndrome* is a condition where microcephaly and body anomalies including short stature, clindactyly of the toes, and genital, facial, and cardiac anomalies. *Rubinstein-Taybi syndrome* is associated with microcephaly, short stature, and developmental delays. The hallmark of this condition is broad thumbs and toes. They also have facial anomalies. *Beckwith's syndrome* is associated with microcephaly and developmental delays. Individuals afflicted with this condition have hypoglycemia in the neonatal period, hemi or focal hypertrophies, umbilical hernias, and characteristic facies.

Seckel's bird-headed dwarf is an autosomal recessive condition associated with retardation, microcephaly, and dwarfism.[72] The individuals afflicted with this condition have bird-like features, low set ears, clubbed feet, and multiple skeletal deformities. *Menke's kinky hair disease* is a sex-linked recessive condition associated with abnormal copper metabolism.[197] Individuals afflicted with Menke's syndrome have short stature, developmental delays, and the hallmark of the condition, fractured stubby friable hair. These individuals have progressive deterioration and progressively severe uncontrollable seizure disorder.

Acquired

Neurotoxic processes that affect the fetus during gestation may be responsible for producing a congenital form of microcephaly. Individuals afflicted with these conditions usually do not show the sloping forehead of the constitutional forms of microcephaly but a globular small head. Processes such as *intrauterinely acquired infections, radiation,* and *hypoxia* may be responsible for producing microcephaly secondary to maldevelopment of the brain (Chapter 3).[53, 46, 47, 106] *Toxic factors* have been shown to produce microcephaly and developmental delays. The ingestion of large amounts of *alcohol* by mothers during pregnancy may result in the fetal alcohol syndrome in the child which produces characteristic midfacial hypoplasia, may produce microcephaly and developmental delays along with other minor congenital anomalies.[198] *Hormonal factors,* specifically uncontrollable diabetes during gestation, may be responsible for producing microcephaly.[68]

Insults to the nervous system *during the perinatal period* may be responsible for producing microcephaly.[47, 106] Primary neurotoxic processes such as *meningoencephalitis* may cause this difficulty.[199] *Hypoxia* is probably the most common cause of neurotoxic insults to the neonate that result in microcephaly (Chapter 4).[106] Individuals who have perinatally acquired microcephaly secondary to insults such as hypoxia often show diffuse cortical atrophy with diminution of white matter producing *hydrocephalus ex vacuo* (large ventricles that fill spaces left by atrophic cortex). In addition, one may also see multiple cystic areas within the brain substance. There are some *viral infections,* particularly herpes simplex type II, which produces a sclerosing encephalitis in the newborn and may be responsible for large cystic cavity production within the cortex, brain atrophy, and resultant microcephaly.[200]

Aberrant Cranial Configurations

Aberrations in head shape often result from premature synostosis of one or more of the cranial sutures.[201] Premature synostosis of sutures will not produce a defect in brain development provided the underlying brain is normal, unless all of the cranial sutures are prematurely synostosed.[202] The brain will expand in areas where there is no premature synostosis. Often there are familial forms of premature cranial synostosis, particularly of the sagittal suture, which are benign conditions. The defects that are produced by simple premature synostosis may affect the cosmetics of the head, but not the function of the brain. In Table VII, there is a list of abnormal head configurations often seen with various premature suture synostoses.

There are certain conditions that are associated with premature synostosis and represent definite syndromes. There are a series of craniofacial dysostosis syndromes where there are premature closures of one or more cranial sutures and malformation of some facial bones.[72, 160, 161] *Crouzon's disease* is the most common of these conditions. This is an autosomal dominant condition where there may be associated developmental disabilities. Individuals afflicted with Crouzon's disease do have facial

Table VII
ABNORMAL CEPHALIC CONFIGURATIONS

Term	Description	Associated Suture Synostosis
Scaphocephaly	long narrow head	sagittal
Dolicocephaly	long narrow head	saggital
Brachycephaly	wide short	unilateral coronal
Acrocephaly	wide conical	bilateral coronal
Plagiocephaly	frontal and contralateral occipital areas flattened	unilateral coronal
Oxycephaly	high pointed	saggital and bilateral coronal
Turricephaly	high pointed	saggital and bilateral coronal
Trigonencephaly	narrow triangular	metopic

abnormalities as well as premature synostosis of their sutures. They have shallow orbits, proptotic eyes, beaked noses, hypoplastic mandible, short upper lips, and protruding lower lips. Individuals may also have proptosis, external strabismus, and maxillary hypoplasia. *Apert's syndrome* is another form of craniofacial dysostosis in which syndactyly of the hands and feet is seen. This is an autosomal dominant condition with an increased incidence of developmental delay. *Carpenter's syndrome* is an autosomal recessive form of craniofacial dysostosis, which is associated with polydactyly (increased number of fingers or toes). Also, there may be syndactyly and mental retardation.

External factors may also be influential in producing abnormalities of head configurations. Infants who lie flat in bed for prolonged periods of time because of neglect or because of hypotonia will develop a flat occiput. Children with developmental disabilities who have delayed motor development may develop a flattening of the occiput. Infants who are left in one position and are unable to freely move from that position may have a flattening of a posterior portion of their cranium. This may lead to plagiocephaly with contralateral bulging of the frontal area. Plagiocephaly is occasionally seen in individuals with or without developmental delays who have torticollis where their head is tilted to one side because of pathology in the sternocleidomastoid muscles (muscles that turn the head from side to side).[201]

Frontal bossing or increased thickening of the frontal bone is a condition that may be a normal variant but may be seen with conditions such as orbital hematomas, tumors, hydranencephaly, and rickets. Individuals may have prominent occiputs that may be a normal variant, a sign of a breech delivery or a sign of Dandy-Walker anomaly. Prominent temporal areas are seen occasionally with neurofibromatosis (Appendix C). Prominent temporal areas may also reflect localized intercranial masses such as tumors, cysts, or hamartomas. Localized bulges may be seen anywhere in the scalp and reflect some underlying pathology such as bony exostosis, encephaloceles, cephalohematomas, arachnoid cysts, or calcified subperiosteal or subgaleal blood.[174]

Chapter 6

SEIZURES

Seizures (epilepsy, convulsions) have been a documented illness of man since the early recorded history.[203] Every individual's nervous system has the potential for having seizures.[204] We all inherit a natural threshold to having seizures. Fortunately, most of us have a sufficiently high threshold so that during our lifetime we do not experience a seizure at any time. However, some individuals have a genetically determined lower threshold[204] and other individuals have had some neurotoxic insult that has lowered their natural threshold either diffusely or in some focal area.[205] Stimuli that can provoke even normal individuals to have seizures include raising the body temperature high enough fast enough, sufficient electrical shock (as used in electrical convulsive therapy), or insulin shock.[204]

Benign febrile seizures are seen in children from the ages of six months to three years of age.[206, 207] At times, it is difficult to distinguish what is a benign febrile seizure and what is a seizure that has been triggered by fever. Febrile seizures by definition are brief (up to five minutes), generalized seizures that do not originate from a focus. They are not associated with a postseizure (Todd's) paralysis. They are associated with an elevated body temperature, and the EEG should return to normal within two weeks after the seizure has occurred. Approximately 4 percent of normal children will have at least one benign febrile seizure before the age of five.[208] Any deviation in character of the seizure from the above-mentioned criteria make one suspicious that the child has an underlying seizure disorder that is being unmasked by fever.[210] Today, most physicians would not treat benign febrile seizures with barbiturate anticonvulsant medication unless the patient has experienced more than two of these episodes or has neurological deficits.[211] Some physicians would wait until the child has experienced multiple episodes before starting him on therapy. Maintenance barbiturate therapy, which produces a blood level within the therapeutic range (see Table VIII), will usually prevent the recurrence of febrile seizures.[212]

Much emphasis has been placed on the EEG for the evaluation of the person with a seizure disorder or with the question of a seizure disorder. Electroencephalograms only record brain electrical activity over thirty minutes or some small fraction of a day. Seizures are paroxysmal events that do not occur even on a daily basis. They occur spontaneously, and a paroxysmal abnormality may not be recorded on the electroencephalogram during the brief period of the tracing.[213] Studies done on patients with documented seizure disorder have shown that 25 percent of individuals with documented seizures will have between two to three normal EEG's.[214] Also, studies in populations of normal individuals have shown that 3 to 5 percent of the population without neurological disease will have some abnormality on their EEG.[215] Electroencephalograms can be helpful in confirming one's clinical impression and also helpful to follow the progress of a patient with a seizure disorder. They may give one clues that the patient could be developing other specific seizure types. Electroencephalograms should not be considered definitive diagnostic tests, but should be used as an aid for diagnosis, treatment, and follow-up.

Most convulsions are of brief duration.[23] They terminate spontaneously, usually before the person can be brought to medical attention. In a person with a documented seizure disorder, the seizure should be permitted to run its course. Medical

Table VIII
THERAPEUTIC BLOOD LEVELS FOR ANTICONVULSANTS

Phenobarbital:	15-40 μgm/ml
Phenytoin:	10-20 μgm/ml
Carbamazepine:	6-12 μmg/ml
Mephobarbital:	Reported as phenobarbital.
Primidone:	5-10 μgm/ml (Note that approximately 30% of primidone is converted to phenobarbital and would be reported as such.)
Valproic Acid:	50-100 μgm/ml
Clonazepam:	30-60 μgm/ml
Ethosuximide:	40-100 μgm/ml

advice need only be sought if the seizure is of longer duration than previous ones, if it has a character that is different from the previous seizures, if the post-ictal (post seizure) state is different in character from that previously seen, or if the patient is having an increase in frequency of his seizures.

Should the person have repetitive major motor seizures without regaining consciousness for a period of over thirty minutes, this is known as status epilepticus.[216] Status epilepticus should be considered an emergency and medical attention sought. The treatment for the patient who is in status is directed towards two goals: (1) the general care of the patient and (2) the administration of appropriate anticonvulsant therapy to terminate the seizures.[23]

Unfortunately, during the acute phase of the seizure, the supportive measures that are so important to the patient are often overlooked. This may even be true in emergency rooms or in hospital situations where medical teams are working on a patient to control his status. There are some very simple, very worthwhile maneuvers that can be performed to help the patient, to prevent the patient from further harm or damage during his seizure. The old measure of prying open clenched teeth with a tongue blade really has no place in the treatment of seizures today. It actually may be harmful, in that it is possible for a person to dislodge or fracture teeth and for the person having the seizure to aspirate his tooth. The tongue biting with a seizure usually occurs in the early tonic phase of the seizure and during that point, when the teeth are clenched down, it is exceptionally difficult if not impossible to pry open the individual's teeth without fracturing them. The old fear that a person will swallow his tongue is really unfounded. To date, a documented case of an individual with normal anatomy who has swallowed his tongue during a seizure has not been reported.[23]

There are some maneuvers that involve common sense and can be quite supportive to a patient experiencing a seizure. Tight clothing especially about the neck should be loosened or removed. The patient's body should be protected against injury caused by extremities involuntarily moving; hard objects should be cleared from the patient's area. Attention should be paid to soft pillows or blankets around the patient; they should be removed to prevent the patient from submerging his head and experiencing hypoxia. If the patient is in a hospital setting, a small plastic airway should be placed into his mouth and taped to his face to provide a patent airway. In the hospital setting, suction should be used to remove excessive saliva, mucus, or vomitus.

Positioning of the patient is very important. Unconscious patients should be turned frequently and patients having a seizure should be allowed to lie on their sides so that saliva, vomitus, and mucus may be drained by gravity from their mouths. Patients should not be allowed to lie supine because of the danger that body fluids may pool in the pharynx and be aspirated into the lungs. Should the patient experience cyanosis during the spell, oxygen should be administered by mask. If the patient is in a hospital setting, his vital signs should be monitored and good supportive nursing care administered.

There is tremendous importance in the administration of supportive maneuvers to a patient having a seizure or in status. It is not the abnormal electrical discharge in the adult that has been implicated as being responsible for further brain damage, but the secondary effects of the autonomic nervous system instability associated with seizures. The particular autonomic nervous system dysfunctions that may lead to further neuronal cell damage include the potential neurotoxic conditions of hyperpyrexia, hypoglycemia, arterial hypotension, and hypoxia.[23]

There are many different drug regimens for the treatment of seizures and for the treatment of status epilepticus.[23, 216-218] The treating physician should be comfortable with a certain set of drugs whose effects and side effects are well known to him. Anticonvulsants should be applied in a systematic manner. The patient or his family should be made aware of the effects and side effects of the anticonvulsant medication utilized. The remainder of the chapter will be devoted to the discussion of seizure types and the medications that are most efficacious for their treatments (see Table IX).[23, 217] Only commonly encountered or potentially acutely life-threatening side effects will be discussed below. For more detailed discussion of side effects, a textbook of pharmacology[219] or the *Physician's Desk Reference* should be consulted.

Table IX
TYPES OF SEIZURE DISORDERS AND THEIR TREATMENT*

I. Major motor seizures.
   A. Grand mal.
      1. Phenobarbital: 4-6 mg/kg/24 hrs (more than 25 kg, give 150 mg/m²) (infants may require higher dosage).
      2. Phenytoin: 4-6 mg/kg/24 hrs (infants may require higher dosage).
      3. Primidone: 10-25 mg/kg/24 hrs.
      4. Mephobarbital: 6-12 mg/kg/24 hrs.
      5. Carbamazepine: 20-25 mg/kg/24 hrs (not approved for use under 6 years).
   B. Status epilepticus.
      1. Phenobarbital: 6 mg/kg (more than 25 kg, give 150 mg/m²) I.M. stat; may repeat times one; may be given I.V.
      2. Diazepam: 0.25 mg/kg I.V. over 5-10 minutes; monitor heart rate and respiration rate; titrate with patient (when patient stops seizure, stop administration).
      3. Amobarbital: 5 mg/kg I.V. (more than 25 kg, give 125 mg/m²) (same precautions as diazepam).
      4. Phenytoin: 15-20 mg/kg I.V. over 30-60 minutes (no faster than 50 mg/min).
      5. After status controlled: Phenobarbital 6 mg/kg q8h times 2 doses, then 4 mg/kg q8h times 3 doses, then maintenance.
II. Massive infantile spasms: ACTH 40 units aqueous q.d. I.M. or 80 units gel q.o.d. I.M.
III. Minor motor seizures.
   A. Mixed minor motor or any of the individual types.
      1. Clonazepam: 0.1-0.2 mg/kg/24 hrs (up to 0.4 mg/kg/24 hrs in selected cases) (must start at 0.025-0.05 mg/kg/24 hrs and gradually increase with careful assessment of clinical signs of drowsiness).
      2. Valproic acid: 20-30 mg/kg/24 hrs (must start at less than 15 mg/kg/24 hrs and gradually increase with careful assessment of clinical signs of drowsiness).
   B. Petit mal.
      1. Ethosuximide: 20-40 mg/kg/24 hrs.
      2. Acetazolamide: 15-30 mg/kg/24 hrs.
   C. Myoclonic seizures.
      1. Diazepam: 0.5-2 mg/kg/24 hrs.
      2. Primidone: 10-20 mg/kg/24 hrs.
   D. Akinetic (see grand mal).
IV. Psychomotor.
   A. Phenytoin: 4-6 mg/kg/24 hrs.
   B. Primidone: 10-25 mg/kg/24 hrs.
   C. Carbamazepine: 20-25 mg/kg/24 hrs.
V. Focal (see grand mal).
VI. Seizure equivalents and borderline epilepsy (see grand mal).

* These are average dosage ranges and clinical signs, individual variations, and serum levels may dictate deviations from them.

Grand Mal

Grand mal seizures are generalized seizures. They can be preceded by an aura or warning. They are characterized by a sudden loss of consciousness. The individual may have tonic and/or clonic movements of muscles of his body. Tonic movements are movements of stiffening where the muscles of one limb, several limbs or the entire body will stiffen usually in extension. Clonic movements are alternating flexion and extension involuntary movements of different muscle groups, usually involving one limb or several limbs. The most common pattern of the grand mal seizure is for the individual to have a brief tonic phase (stiffening) followed by a more prolonged clonic phase (muscles alternately flexing and extending). After the episode terminates, it may be followed by a period of post-ictal (post seizure) drowsiness or sleep. Grand mal seizures are the most common of all seizure types. There are several medications that are effective in treating grand mal seizures.

Phenobarbital

Phenobarbital is an excellent anticonvulsant for the treatment of grand mal seizures. It is one of the oldest of the anticonvulsants in common usage today. The dosage of phenobarbital as for most anticonvulsants depends upon body weight or surface area. One would use 4 to 6 mg/kg/24 hours in individuals less than 25 kg and 150 mg/m^2 in individuals over 25 kg. Phenobarbital should be divided into a three times a day dose schedule for infants and into a twice a day dose schedule for young children. Many adolescents and adults are able to tolerate phenobarbital on a once a day dose schedule. The side effects of phenobarbital are relatively few with skin rashes occasionally seen as a manifestation of an allergy. Much has been written concerning behavioral changes associated with phenobarbital. There is some controversy in the literature as to the frequency of patients on phenobarbital therapy having behavioral disorders or hyperactivity. It is not uncommon for children who are placed on phenobarbital to become hyperactive or to have some behavioral change for the first seven to fourteen days of treatment, but this often will abate. However, permanent hyperactivity reactions may occur. Another side effect of phenobarbital is somnolence, drowsiness, and ataxia. Occasionally this will pass within seven to fourteen days but beyond that period of time it is often dose related. Should the person have too high a dosage of phenobarbital, drowsiness, ataxia and somnolence can be experienced. If a person is getting *exceedingly* high doses of phenobarbital, respiratory depression, coma and even death may occur. However, these side effects are seen only in exceedingly high doses of medication.

Phenytoin (Dilantin®)

Phenytoin is another very good anticonvulsant for treating grand mal seizures. The dosage is 4 to 6 mg/kg/24 hours. Phenytoin as Dilantin® has the benefit of being given in a once a day dosage at any age level. When it is administered in a maintenance dose schedule it will take up to two weeks to achieve a therapeutic circulating blood level. Therefore, many individuals who start a patient on Dilantin will "Dilantinize" the patient by giving high dosage of the medication for one to three days as an initial loading period. There are many reported side effects of Dilantin. One that is not uncommonly seen is gingival hypertrophy (overgrowth of the gums). This is often seen in individuals with developmental disabilities who have poor dental hygiene and who tend to chew the Dilantin in tablet form. There are some clinicians who feel that good dental hygiene and the use of Dilantin capsules may lessen or prevent the occurrence of gingival hypertrophy. Another side effect is skin rash as a manifestation of allergy, which may progress to severe exfoliative dermatitis. Chemical hepatitis has been reported. Hematopoietic disturbances have also been shown to occur particularly with a drop in white blood cell count. In addition, hyperplasia of the lymphoid tissue and even lymphoma have been reported. Other minor side effects would include hirsuitism (excessive hairiness) and soft tissue overgrowth. There has been reported a higher incidence of rickets and osteomalacia (decalcification of bone) in patients receiving anticonvulsant therapy particularly those receiving therapy with Dilantin. It is therefore advisable that individuals who are placed on Dilantin or other anticonvulsants receive treatment with vitamin D. Although the dosage has not been totally agreed upon, the dosage of between 200 and 500 units of vitamin D per day is generally used. There are some individuals on phenytoin who may experience a situation where there is a vitamin D resistant rickets and one should be on the alert for the occurrence of pathological fractures in patients receiving phenytoin therapy, particularly those who are bedridden. Phenytoin as well as any other anticonvulsant in excessive dosages can make a patient ataxic or somnolent. It is exceedingly difficult for a patient to take a sufficient overdosage to cause coma and death.

Primidone (Mysoline®)

Primidone is an anticonvulsant of the barbiturate type. One third of it is metabolized to phenobarbital in order to become therapeutically active. The dosage of primidone is 10 to 25 mg/kg/24 hours. The side effects are similar to that of the barbiturate phenobarbital. When one uses primidone as an anticonvulsant it should be spaced into a b.i.d. or t.i.d. dose schedule regardless of age. Some individuals when first starting on primidone may become ataxic or somnolent and they may require starting at a very low dosage, gradually increasing until their therapeutic dose schedule is reached over several days.

Mephobarbital (Mebaral®)

Mephobarbital is another anticonvulsant in the barbiturate class. It is converted 100 percent to phenobarbital to be therapeutically active. The dose schedule is 6 to 12 mg/kg/24 hours. In general it is administered in a b.i.d. or t.i.d. dose schedule. The side effects seen in mephobarbital are similar to that seen with phenobarbital. It is interesting to note however that the side effect of hyperactivity or behavioral disturbance is rarely reported with mephobarbital (and primidone) in contrast to phenobarbital. This is interesting from the standpoint that all of mephobarbital is converted to phenobarbital and a third of primidone is converted to phenobarbital. This phenomenon may reflect the expectation of behavioral changes with phenobarbital. True hyperactivity reactions have occurred with all of the barbiturates.

Carbamazepine (Tegretol®)

Carbamazepine is administered in dosage of 20 to 25 mg/kg/ 24 hours. The average adult dosage is 1200 mg; the maximum recommended dosage is 1600 mg per day. It is usually divided into a twice a day or three times a day dose schedule. This medication has not been released for use by the FDA in children under six years of age. However, there are some studies reporting its use in young children with good results and without excessive side effects. The side effects of concern are an alteration of the hematopoietic system with a diminution of white cells, red cells, and platelets and also the occurrence of chemical hepatitis. It is for this reason that frequent blood counts and liver function studies are recommended for individuals on carbamazepine therapy. Other side effects would be renal dysfunction, skin rash, and, in excessive doses, ataxia and somnolence.

Status Epilepticus

Status epilepticus is the frequent recurrence of generalized seizures between which the patient does not regain consciousness. The episode must last for a minimum of thirty minutes to be classified as status epilepticus.[216] Status epilepticus is a serious event and is a neurological emergency. One study done on children in status epilepticus showed that 11 percent of the children died in status with 6 percent of the total dying in status without any other cause. In addition, 19 percent of the individuals who had normal neurological examinations prior to going into status epilepticus had neurological abnormalities after the event.[220] There are many different treatment regiments for status epilepticus, but the treatment must extend beyond simply stopping the status. The patient should be placed on high doses of medication in hospital until he is totally stabilized.

Phenobarbital (Luminal®)

Phenobarbital is often used in the treatment of status epilepticus. The initial dose is between 6 and 20 mg/kg as a starting dose. If the individual is over 25 kg, the usual starting dose is 150 mg/m^2. One advantage of phenobarbital is that it can be effectively used intramuscularly as well as intravenously in status epilepticus. If one started with a 6 mg/kg dose or 150 mg/m^2, it could be repeated in fifteen minutes if the status epilepticus has not ceased.

Diazepam (Valium®)

Diazepam is a drug that can be used to stop status epilepticus in the acute situation. However, it is only efficacious for approximately fifteen to twenty minutes in controlling seizures so that after the seizure activity has been stopped with diazepam, the patient should be treated with other anticonvulsants for maintenance therapy. The average dose of diazepam in children is 0.1 to 0.2 mg/kg, and it should be administered only intravenously. In adults the average starting dose is 10 mg. This medication for the treatment of status should be administered with caution. It should be given slowly (five to ten minutes) with the heart rate and respiratory rate monitored. Medication should be administered until the seizure activity stops. At that point, no further medication need be given even if the full dosage has not been administered.

Paraldehyde

Paraldehyde is a medication that can be used in the treatment of status epilepticus and can be given by the rectal, nasogastric, or intravenous route. For intravenous use, 10 cc of paraldehyde is mixed with 200 ml of glucose water. It is then given to the patient by intravenous drip and the patient's seizures titrated with paraldehyde administration. Unfortunately, paraldehyde has the side effect of being excreted by the lung. Hence, the patient will emit a rather pungent odor when treated with paraldehyde. The general starting dose is 0.2 cc of paraldehyde concentrate per kilogram.

Phenytoin (Dilantin®)

Phenytoin has recently come into use for the treatment of status epilepticus. The dosage is 15 to 30 mg/kg. It is administered intravenously over thirty to sixty minutes (maximum rate 50 mg/min). During the administration of the phenytoin the patient's heart rate must be monitored because of the side effect of ventricular arrhythmia, which can be life threatening.

Valproic Acid (Depakene®)

Recently valproic acid has been used in the treatment of status epilepticus. The dosage ranges between 200 to 600 mg every six hours for the first day. It should be administered by nasogastric tube or by rectal suppository. (For more information on valproic acid see section on minor motor seizures below). After the first twenty-four hours of treatment, valproic acid maintenance therapy can be begun at 30 to 50 mg/kg/24 hours divided into q8h dosage.[221]

After the status epilepticus is controlled, the patient must be maintained on high doses of anticonvulsants for several days. One such regimen would include treatment with phenobarbital 6 mg/kg (150 mg/m^2 if greater than 25 kg) every 8 hours × 2 doses, then 4 mg/kg q8h (100 mg/m^2 if greater than 25 kg) for 3 doses and on the third day, put the patient on maintenance phenobarbital.

Massive Infantile Spasms

Massive infantile spasms are known by a variety of other names in the literature including West's syndrome, salaam seizures, infantile myoclonus, or infantile spasms. These seizures characteristically occur in the age bracket of three months to three years with the average age of onset in the six to twelve month age range. It is unusual to see these seizures after three years of age, and they are almost never seen after five years of age. Massive infantile spasms are characterized by sudden transient contraction of the limbs and/or head and/or trunk. They last only for a second. They may occur in a cluster. They often occur when the child is somnolent or drowsy. These seizures in and of themselves do not interfere with the child's normal random baby activity. Oftentimes, before the onset of the massive infantile spasms, the child who has had a normal disposition will be excessively irritable. At times, when the child is having a spasm, he may briefly cry out.

Massive infantile spasms are a devastating problem, because even with treatment, only 20 to 30 percent of afflicted children will have an intelligence in the normal range (IQ greater than 80). Children with this affliction fall into two categories. Those who have infantile spasms as a symptom of another underlying disease such as post-hypoxic encephalopathy, encephalitis, certain aminoacidopathies, tuberosclerosis, etc., and those who fall into cryptogenic (idiopathic) categories, in whom no prior disease state can be found. In general, children who fall into the cryptogenic group do better than children who fall into the symptomatic group in terms of their ultimate outcome. Other factors that predict a better outcome are the early initiation of treatment after the onset of spasms and a normal development up until the time the child develops the massive infantile spasms.[222]

Massive infantile spasms are associated with an abnormal pattern on EEG called hypsarrhthmia (multiple independent spikes occurring in all recording leads and one to two cycles per second high voltage slowing). The treatment for massive infantile spasms is steroid hormones. Although any number of steroids may be employed for treatment of massive infantile spasms, it appears that the best results are achieved with a long course of ACTH. The recommended dose schedule would be 40 units of ACTH every day intramuscularly or subcutaneously.[222] There is no uniform agreement as to how long to put the patient on therapy or what constitutes the total daily dose. It is often useful to treat the patient with a minimum of three months time. With treatment, most patients will have a cessation of their spasms and a reversion of their EEG to a nonhypsarrhythmic pattern, although the EEG usually remains abnormal. The patient who is treated with steroid hormones should gradually have his medication tapered over a period of months. During the period of tapering, the patient should be watched closely for the recredescence of the massive infantile spasms or the abnormal hypsarrhythmic pattern on the EEG.

MIXED MINOR MOTOR SEIZURES

Mixed minor motor seizures are a phenomena that often have their onset at the age range of three to six years. Many children who have massive infantile spasms will progress in time to develop mixed minor motor seizures. This type of seizure's manifestations are, as the name implies, minor but also motor in character. They may consist of any of the traditional forms of minor motor seizures such as petit mal or akinetic and myoclonic jerks (defined below), but also may take on the character of any minor repetitive motor act.[223, 224] Many of these seizures would appear much like the subtle seizure of the infant (Chapter 4). Very often these children will have acts that appear brief and repetitive and stereotyped. Occasionally, casual observers may feel that this has just been part of the child's behavior pattern when it may represent seizure activity.

Often with mixed minor motor seizures one sees a rather characteristic pattern on EEG. This is called a Lennox-Gestaut pattern and consists of atypical 3 cps spike and slow waves. The occurrence of mixed minor motor seizures, retardation, and the Lennox-Gastaut pattern on EEG is known as the Lennox-Gastaut triad. Until recently, there were no medications that were uniformly therapeutically effective against this devastating seizure problem. Two new medications have been developed that have a high success rate in treating mixed minor motor seizures or any form of minor motor seizure activity. These medications are clonazepam and valproic acid.

Clonazepam (Clonopin®)

Clonazepam[225-228] is a medication that is related to diazepam (Valium®) in structure. It is usually prescribed in a dose range of 0.1-0.2 mg/kg/24 hours. This is divided into a 3 times a day or 4 times a day dose schedule. At times it is necessary to increase the dosage to 0.4 mg/kg/24 hours. One of the major side effects of clonazepam therapy is somnolence which usually occurs when starting a patient on this medication. Therefore, it is recommended that patients be started on a very low dosage of the medication, 0.025-0.05 mg/kg/24 hours and increases of an absolute amount of 0.5 mg every 3 to 7 days be undertaken until the maintenance dose schedule is achieved. The side effects of clonazepam except for the drowsiness are relatively minor but include skin rashes, increase in appetite and behavior disturbances.

Valproic Acid (Depakene®)

Valproic acid[229-231] is another medication that is useful in the treatment of mixed minor motor seizure disorders. The usual daily dosage for this medication is 30 mg/kg/24 hours divided into a three or four times a day dose schedule. In some individuals it may be necessary to increase the dose to 60 mg/kg/24 hours. Again, this medication may induce somnolence and ataxia when initially started. Therefore, it is recommended that most individuals who start on the medication begin on a daily dose schedule of 15 mg/kg/24 hours and that the medication be gradually increased by 5 mg/kg/24 hours every three to seven days until maintenance dosages are achieved. Although initially thought to be an exceedingly safe as well as efficacious medication, there are more side effects being reported with valproic acid therapy. Some of the most serious include chemical hepatitis and alterations of the hematopoietic system, particularly diminution in platelet number or platelet effectiveness. (Platelets are the blood element which enables our blood to clot when necessary.) Other side effects that have been observed with valproic acid would include nausea and vomiting, transitory hair loss, pancreatitis,[232] tremors,[233] allergic skin rashes, and renal dysfunction.

Petit Mal

Petit mal seizures are a very distinctive seizure type. They are a form of minor motor seizure. It is important to emphasize that the term *petit mal* does *not* refer to brief grand mal or partial major motor seizure. Petit mal seizures are brief lapses of consciousness characterized by vacant staring of the eyes during which purposeful movements cease. There may be some rhythmical movements of the lips, eyelids, and fingertips, but most individuals would not accept changes in postural tone as a manifestation of petit mal seizures. Each episode lasts for a matter of seconds but clearly less than thirty seconds. The episodes may occur up to several hundreds of times a day. Petit mal seizures characteristically occur in the four to twelve year age range. It is interesting to note that a certain percentage, approximately 30 to 40 percent of children afflicted with petit mal seizures, will have petit mal only for a transient period in their life and never be troubled again with seizure disorders. However, most individuals who have petit mal will have other seizure types in addition to the petit mal or, when the petit mal abates, will progress to other forms of seizures. Although clonazepam and valproic acid may be used to treat this seizure disorder, the drug of choice for treatment of petit mal seizures is ethosuximide.

Ethosuximide (Zarontin®)

Ethosuximide is administered in a dose schedule of 20 to 40 mg/kg/24 hours and should be administered in a twice a day or three times a day dose schedule. This drug is a safe medication. The only frequently observed side effect of ethosuximide therapy is nausea which may occur at the time the medication is administered. Should this occur, it may be necessary to give the medication with meals. However, in some children, nausea may persist and it would be necessary to choose another medication. Other side effects include allergic skin reactions, hematopoietic or hepatic disturbance.

Acetazolamide (Diamox®)

This medication is no longer considered a first line drug in the treatment of petit mal seizures. However, it can be efficacious as a second drug for petit mal or for other seizure disorders as well. Acetazolamide has its effect by altering the pH. It is often useful for females who have their seizures (major motor type) primarily around the time of menses, as an additional medication. The dose of azetazolamide is 15 to 30 mg/kg/24 hours and it should be divided into a b.i.d. or t.i.d. dose schedule.

Myoclonic Seizures

Myoclonic seizures are sudden involuntary contractions of large muscle groups about the limbs or the face or the trunk. During the myoclonic seizure there is no apparent loss of consciousness. The medications that can be used to treat myoclonic seizures in addition to valproic acid and clonazepam would include diazepam and primidone. The dose of diazepam would be

0.5 to 2 mg/kg/24 hours. This medication may induce somnolence and the dosage should be begun at a low level and increased until maintenance is reached.

Akinetic Seizures

Akinetic seizures are characterized by a transient loss of postural tone and a sudden fall or drop. The individual may lose consciousness as he is falling. If he does lose consciousness, he will awaken immediately upon falling. In addition to valproic acid and clonazepam, the medications used to treat akinetic spells are those used to treat grand mal seizures.

PSYCHOMOTOR SEIZURES

Psychomotor seizures (temporal lobe, partial complex) are protean in their manifestations. Their manifestations can include mental, motor, or sensory symptoms. They may be characterized by sudden periods of vacant staring lasting minutes or hours, periods of complex hallucinations, sudden alterations of consciousness, drowsy dreamlike states, periods of automatic uncontrolled behavior, periods of autonomic nervous system dysfunction such as lip smacking, eyelid fluttering, periods of aphasia, periods of inappropriate flow of words, or periods of quasipurposeful activities. Temporal lobe seizures are at times exceedingly difficult to diagnose because their manifestations are so varied. It is often difficult to discern temporal lobe seizures from behavioral disorders in individuals. To complicate matters, approximately 16 percent of individuals who have temporal lobe seizures have a temporal lobe personality that is an antisocial hostile aggressive personality type.[23] An aid to making this diagnosis is the occurrence of an abnormal EEG, particularly one that shows dysfunction in one or both temporal lobes. However, abnormal EEG's are only seen in approximately 80 percent of individuals with temporal lobe seizure disorders.[213] Temporal lobe seizures are a frequently encountered seizure type in older children and adolescents. It is entirely possible that an individual may not have any manifestations of seizures until they become pubescent, when temporal lobe seizures may become manifested. They do occur in younger children, but not with a frequency that they occur in older children and adolescents.

The reason that the temporal lobe seizures are so varied in their manifestations and may involve so many behavioral or repetitive motor acts in their manifestation relates to the unique position of the temporal lobe in the nervous system. It is the portion of our brain that is in close proximity and in intimate connection with the portions of our nervous system that control our emotions, control our behavior, and also control our autonomic nervous system function. The relatively high frequency with which temporal lobe seizure disorders occur may relate to the unique physiologic aspects of the temporal lobe. Specific neuronal cell groups within the temporal lobe are highly vulnerable to hypoxia and are often damaged and/or destroyed by hypoxic insults. Also, the unique position of the temporal lobe (sitting within a bony cavity at the lower portion of the calvarium) makes it vulnerable to injury with head trauma and during birth. The temporal lobe has both cells that are particularly vulnerable to injury and an anatomical position that is particularly vulnerable to injury. The medications of choice in treating temporal lobe seizures would be phenytoin and carbamazepam. Primidone and phenobarbital are also effective.

FOCAL SEIZURES

When individuals think of focal seizures they usually think of the focal motor Jacksonian seizure that is a specific type of focal motor seizure beginning as a march, starting with the thumb, progressing to the hand, to the arm and the face and the leg and finally becoming generalized. Focal motor seizures do not all follow this Jacksonian pattern. They may involve simply a finger, hand, or leg without having a characteristic march. In addition to focal motor seizures, focal seizures can also take on sensory characteristics or visual phenomena. Focal seizures in adolescents and adults usually point to some structural lesion in the area of the brain that is involved. For example, focal sensory seizures often reflect parietal lobe damage. Focal visual phenomena of flashing lights may reflect occipital lobe disease and focal hallucinatory phenomena may reflect temporal lobe disease. In infants, focal seizures do not have the same localizing significance as they have in adults. Treatment for focal seizures whether they are motor, sensory, visual or hallucinatory would be the same as for grand mal epilepsy.

BORDERLINE EPILEPSY

There are several conditions that could be classified as autonomic seizures or borderline epilepsy. Phenomena such as paroxysmal abdominal pain, cyclic vomiting, episodic dizziness, periodic headaches, episodic inappropriate laughter, etc., may be seizures. It is often difficult to prove that these phenomena are seizures except the use of a clinical trial with one of the grand mal anticonvulsant medications. The purpose of the clinical trial is to determine if the symptom will be abated by the use of anticonvulsant medication. It would be confirmatory to one's clinical impression if the EEG were abnormal. Anticonvulsants used to treat the autonomic seizures would be the grand mal medications.

GENERAL COMMENTS

When managing a patient with a seizure disorder it is best to start with only one medication and then to take that medication to the upper limits of its normal therapeutic range. Over the past decade, the use of serum levels for anticonvulsant therapy has come into the foreground. Table VIII lists the normal therapeutic blood levels for various anticonvulsants.[234, 235] The reader should be aware that the anticonvulsant dosages suggested in Table IX are the average doses that will produce a serum blood level in the average therapeutic range.[217, 234, 235] However, there are many individuals who will require higher dosage or lower dosage to achieve the therapeutic range. Also there are individuals who will be able to tolerate blood levels of anticonvulsants considerably higher than the recommended therapeutic range. Provided the patient is asymptomatic, it is generally not harmful for anticonvulsant levels to be slightly above the therapeutic range. Early signs of intoxication with anticonvulsants are somnolence, ataxia, unsteadiness, nystagmus, and incoordination. If these signs are present, it is often wise to decrease the anticonvulsant dosage.

When treating a patient with a seizure disorder, it is important to realize that the individual may be on medication for an indefinite period of time. Since there are only a few good anticonvulsant choices for each seizure type, it is best to alter therapy slowly in patients who have seizures. Changes should be made one at a time. If one were to add another drug or change drugs, the new drug should be added and, after it has reached a therapeutic level, the old drug should be tapered. If someone were to have an allergic reaction to a medication, it should be stopped immediately and the patient treated with another anticonvulsant.

The length of time it is necessary to maintain a person on anticonvulsants after he is seizure free is not completely agreed upon.[236, 237] If the patient has a simple seizure disorder, many individuals would treat for two to four years seizure free and then consider tapering the patient off medication. However, if the individual has a complicated seizure disorder, one should wait at least four years before discontinuing the anticonvulsant. A complex seizure problem is — (1) one in which the EEG was severely abnormal at the outset and changed little over the years; (2) one where the EEG remains abnormal; (3) a seizure disorder that started after the age of nine years; (4) a seizure disorder that requires more than six years to control; (5) one that required multiple medications in order to achieve control; (6) an individual who has multiple seizure types; (7) a focal or Jacksonian seizure disorder; or (8) an individual with psychological or neurological deficits. In many individuals with severe developmental disabilities, it is often advisable to maintain anticonvulsant medication for an indefinite period of time since they have neurological brain damage.

In general, it is wise to maintain an anticonvulsant treated person on vitamin D since there is an increased incidence of vitamin D dependent rickets in patients treated with anticonvulsants.[238-240] It is often wise to monitor the blood count (CBC) and the liver function (SGOT, SGPT) once a year. If the patient is being treated with medication with known hematopoietic or hepatic dysfunction, e.g. valproic acid, carbamazepine, then these studies should be obtained at more frequent intervals (at least every three months).

Chapter 7

CEREBRAL PALSY

THE TERM *cerebral palsy* refers to a heterogeneous group of conditions characterized by some aberration of motor function caused by pathology in motor control centers of the brain. Clinical manifestations can be quite varied. There can be paralysis, weakness, incoordination, tremor, involuntary movements, rigidity, stiffness, or any aberration in motor function. Cerebral palsy results from an injury or insult that occurs at the time of birth, before birth, or in the immediate perinatal period (first twenty-eight days of life). There are some definitions that would include anyone who receives an injury to his nervous system motor centers during childhood, but a purist definition would include only children who had their insults either prenatally or perinatally.[243, 244]

Cerebral palsy will present a variety of clinical pictures. There is a continuum of involvement from mild to severe. If an insult occurs that damages one part of a nervous system (in this case the motor control centers), other parts of the nervous system could be affected. Many of the children with cerebral palsy with other parts of their nervous system involving intelligence, behavior, activity level, seizures, etc.[245, 246] Of individuals with cerebral palsy, 25 percent have a normal intelligence; 45 percent are moderately or severely retarded; and 30 percent are of borderline intelligence. The incidence of cerebral palsy is two per thousand population.[247]

Since the clinical manifestations of cerebral palsy are so variable, it is important to have a framework with which to communicate information; simply using the term *cerebral palsy* is a nonspecific description of motor dysfunction. A method is needed for classifying and specifically stating the clinical manifestations of cerebral palsy. Descriptive terminology would include the degree, type of disability, and location of the disability.[248, 249]

107

DEGREE

Degree would be qualification on severity of the condition. Patients can be separated into *mild, moderate,* and *severe.* The mildly affected individual would be ambulatory and does not need any special aids to ambulate, but would benefit from some therapy or intervention. The moderately affected individual would have impaired self-help skills, impaired ambulation, and could definitely profit from some treatment modalities. The severely affected individual would be severely incapacitated, definitely need special devices, would not be ambulatory, and may require custodial care. There are further qualifiers that could be applied to further qualify the severity of the condition, e.g. very mild, soft, very severe, etc.

TYPE

The types of disability are varied. The most common type is *spasticity,* and this is the form of cerebral palsy most individuals think about when they hear of cerebral palsy. Spasticity is the tendency of muscles to contract when put under stress. Spastic individuals will have very stiff muscle groups. The stiffness often becomes more severe with time, and they may become contracted down in position further limiting their mobility. They tend to have exaggerated deep tendon reflexes.

Athetoid individuals have purposeless, involuntary, rhythmic, irregular, uncontrollable motions of varying muscle tone. Athetoid movements occur about small muscle groups around small joints. These movements are often seen involving fingers, toes, or facial muscles. This is in contrast to *chorea,* which are purposeless, involuntary, rhythmical, uncontrollable motions. Choreoform movements are coarser and involve larger muscle groups. The distinction between chorea and athetosis is sometimes very difficult, and many individuals have both chorea and athetosis. *Choreoathetotic* individuals have the involuntary movements about the small and large muscle groups.

Rigidity describes individuals who have muscle groups with extreme resistance to passive motion. *Tremor* can be another manifestation of cerebral palsy. Tremor is an uncontrollable, involuntary motion but has a rhythmical, alternating, or pendular quality. Individuals may have *ataxia,* which is a disturbance of imbalance or postural sense.

Hypotonia or *atonia* may be a manifestation of cerebral palsy. Although most individuals do not think of atonia or hypotonia as manifestations of cerebral palsy, this may be a manifestation. There are many children who initially manifest hypotonia or atonia, but may progress to spasticity. It is not uncommon for an initially atonic cerebral palsied child to become spastic over months or years. Many individuals will have more than one problem with their motor system. Eighty to eighty-five percent of individuals with cerebral palsy have more than one type of difficulty in their motor control system.

Location

There are a series of terms that describe the areas of involvement. *Diplegia* is probably the most common location for cerebral palsy. The term *diplegia* means that all four limbs are involved, with the legs involved to a greater extent than the arms. This is in contrast to the term *paraplegia,* which means there is only involvement of the legs and no involvement of the arms. Physiologically it is difficult to have paraplegia on the basis of a brain insult. It is more common on the basis of spinal cord insult. If one is confronted with a child who has paraplegia, one should investigate the spinal column to determine if the pathology is there. The term *double hemiplegia* refers to involvement of all four extremities, but the arms more than the legs. *Hemiplegia* means only one side of the body is involved. *Monoplegia* implies involvement of just one limb. If a child has a monoplegia, one should look closely for pathology at the major plexuses, the brachial plexus or the sacral plexus. Sacral plexus injuries are exceptionally rare, but, in the newborn period, brachial plexus injuries are occasionally seen.

The term *quadriplegia* means involvement of all four extremities to an equal degree. *Triplegia* refers to involvement of three extremities. Physiologically it is difficult to produce triplegia. Most individuals who demonstrate involvement of three extremities represent a diplegia with a superimposed hemiplegia, which would produce involvement of three limbs primarily.

Another localizing term is the *pseudobulbar palsy.* This term may be confusing because of the similar term *pseudobulbar state.* In pseudobulbar state, individuals (primarily adults) may have pseudobulbar palsy but also have inappropriate laughter and crying, a loss of social amenities, and loss of bowel and bladder control. A pseudobulbar palsy refers to pathology in the cortical control centers of the bulbar motor nuclei (controls muscles of the head and neck). The problem in pseudobulbar palsy is not in the bulbar nuclei of the brain stem, but in the cerebral control of these nuclei. Individuals with pseudobulbar palsy can reflexly move these muscle groups, but cannot voluntarily move them smoothly. They may have difficulties with swallowing, tongue movements, sucking movements, speech, etc.[250]

Pathological change in the brain of individuals with cerebral palsy can be quite variable.[251, 252] There may be changes only on a microscopic level, e.g. diminution in number of neurons in areas, pigment staining of certain neurons or increased numbers of glial cells. In many individuals, no abnormalities may be found on gross or microscopic examination. There is some investigative evidence that defective dendritic arborization may relate to the production of developmental disabilities in individuals with grossly normal appearing brains.[122, 253]

The etiology of cerebral palsy is as varied as the agents that can cause neurotoxic insults, e.g. hypoxia, infection, etc. (Chapter 4). Anything that can adversely affect the developing brain can cause cerebral palsy or other developmental disabilities.[244, 252, 254]

Cerebral palsy is not a unitary diagnostic term, but a term referring to varied aberrations of the motor control centers of the brain based on an insult that occurred perinatally or prenatally.

Treatment

There are various modes of treatment for children with cerebral palsy. The child with cerebral palsy is best served with an interdisciplinary team approach since they may have other developmental disabilities in addition to their motor dysfunction. Even if their problem is purely motor, they often require evaluation and treatment by more than one discipline. They may need an orthopedist, an occupational therapist, physical therapist, and neurologist. It is the interdisciplinary team that can call for multiple evaluations and together decide on a uniform approach to these children.

Braces and mechanical aids are treatment modalities that are used for children with cerebral palsy. They are used to prevent deformities, used to stretch contractures, to provide stability for a joint, provide some joint positioning postoperatively, or to control involuntary movements. There are problems with braces and mechanical aids. Children may outgrow them rapidly. They can become malaligned, or ambulatory children may force them out of alignment. One of the potential dangers with bracing and mechanical aids is that the child may rely on them and not strengthen his muscles. These aids are best used in an integrated program of therapy so that muscular atrophy does not occur. *Nighttime casting* may be useful because that is the point at which a child would not be using his limbs and they can be properly positioned for several hours.

Surgery is another mode of therapy that is used.[255] This is often used for spasticity to relieve contractures. Tendon resections are often performed particularly about the heel cord. Muscle transplants may be performed that switch the flexors and extensors about a joint. There are operations for joint stabilization. There can be nerve resections. Regardless of the type of surgery, it is important to plan surgery with other forms of therapy, e.g. bracing and physical therapy.

There are also *medications* that are used primarily to induce relaxation about muscle groups. The two most popular are dantrium sodium and diazepam. These are best used in conjunction with a program of physical therapy. *Physical therapy* and *occupational therapy* should be initiated early, before deformities are apparent. Once a joint has been contracted down it becomes difficult to release contractures by simple therapy. Preventive therapy can prevent the joint contractures and may obviate the need for surgery at a later date.

There are many maneuvers that are used in physical therapy and there are many good schools of thought and different ways of approaching physical therapy in individuals with cerebral palsy. Any form of therapy that alleges to facilitate or hasten development by special maneuvers should be carefully scrutinized.[4, 256, 257] Therapy's aim is to allow the child to achieve his potential and to prevent anything, e.g. spasticity, that would interfere with his developmental progress. There is no physiological way to make a nervous system develop faster than it is destined to develop, regardless of how often or what methods are used to reposture or position the child (Chapter 1). The patient with cerebral palsy may require other forms of specialized therapy, e.g. speech therapy.

The defect in cerebral palsy lies within the confines of the central nervous system, but what is seen on the patient is merely a reflection of the peripheral manifestations of a central nervous system dysfunction. Therapy should be directed toward the prevention of contractures or deformities, to their correction, should they occur, and following their correction, appropriate treatment to prevent their recurrence.

Developmental Approach

In order to put treatment in its proper perspective, it is important to realize that many of the clinical manifestations of cerebral palsy result from developmental lags in gross motor skills.[258] From the developmental viewpoint, cerebral palsy represents a profound deficit in motor and sensory maturation and integration. It is the delay in the acquisition of motor skills and the delay in the progression through normal states in development that leads to the hypertrophy of certain primitive reflexes and, secondarily, to many of the clinical motor manifestations of this disorder. Children with cerebral palsy do not progress at the normal rate through the stages of motor development (see Table I).

Certain postures seen in the child with cerebral palsy can be related to the hypertrophy of certain specific primitive reflexes.[259] Persistence and subsequent hypertrophy of the infantile posture (Figure 2) will produce an increase in flexor tone in the upper extremity. This will become more pronounced the longer the posture persists beyond the zero-to-four week age range; muscles will become contracted down and adduction and flexion in the upper extremity, producing posture commonly seen in infants with spasticity in the upper extremities. The persistence of the infantile posture will lead to flexion contracture of the hand and the persistence of the thumb in the position of the infant, which many individuals label as a cortical thumb. This merely represents the hypertrophy of a primitive body reflex.

In the lower extremities, the persistence and hypertrophy of the positive proprioceptive supporting response (Figure 11) will cause an increase in extension extensor tone and adductor tone of the hip and lower extremities. The positive proprioceptive supporting response will be elicited by pressure either on the balls of the foot or on the buttocks. It is the hypertrophy of this reflex that leads to the increase in extensor tone and adductor tone in the lower extremities commonly seen in individuals with spastic diplegias or spastic quadriplegias. This may lead to toe walking or to scissoring of the gait. In addition, the plantar grasp (Figure 12), which can be stimulated by pressure on the ball of the foot, may hypertrophy, leading to increase in the plantar flexion of the toes. Children who have increase in muscular tone with the hypertrophy of the positive proprioceptive supporting response may have such increased tone in their pelvic girdle and legs that they will stand early but will have difficulty sitting at the appropriate time. They stand when they are placed in a standing position.

A child who has stabilized in the asymmetric tonic neck stage (Figure 3) of development (four weeks to four months) will manifest increased extensor tone on one side of the body and increased flexor tone on the opposite side of the body. This reflex is reinforced when his head is persistently turned to one side.

Some manifestations of difficulty with prehension may also be related to the hypertrophy of certain primitive reflexes.[260-262] In the child who has a persistence and then hypertrophy of the traction response, when he attempts to reach out for objects, placing stretch on the shoulder adductors, he may stimulate this traction response causing the flexion of his fingers and flexion of the joints in that upper extremity. This will produce the appearance of the reflex withdrawal upon reaching for objects. Some children have inability to let go of objects that are placed in their hand. This can be seen in children who have a persistence of hypertrophy of the palmar grasp and contact grasp (Figure 6) where tactile stimuli presented to the palm or hand causes reflex flexion of the fingers.

Some children with cerebral palsy may have difficulty in holding onto objects placed in their hands although they are developmentally mature. This may represent severe developmental lag or may represent a hypertrophy of the avoiding response (Figure 16), which can be stimulated by light touch to the dorsal surface of the hand or if hypertrophied, by pulsed air. Even mild movement of the hand through the air may stimulate the avoiding response causing extension of the fingers and causing the children to drop the object they are holding in their hand.

The visual avoiding response may also be hypertrophied in children with cerebral palsy. This is a natural response that occurs when a threatening stimulus is presented to us. We turn our head and eyes away. In some children with cerebral palsy, this response becomes hypertrophied, and they reflexively visually avoid objects as they approach them whether they be threatening or nonthreatening.

In some children, athetosis may be viewed as the result of the hypertrophy and instability of the interaction between the avoiding response (Figure 16) and the palmar grasp response, so that there is a constant instability between these responses, causing flexion alternating with extension of the muscles about the fingers.

Cerebral palsy is really a heterogeneous group of conditions that relate to an aberration of motor function caused by pathology in motor control centers in the brain. In many instances, the clinical manifestations of the defect results from a hypertrophy and persistence of certain primitive reflexes. Many of the clinical manifestations of children with cerebral palsy may be viewed as a developmental lag or arrest in the acquisition of gross motor skills.

Chapter 8

HYPOTONIA

HYPOTONIA IS A STATE in which the resistance to passive motion of the muscle groups is less than normally anticipated for the child at his chronological age.[263] The symptom of hypotonia in childhood has multiple etiologies.[264] The distinction between upper motor neuron lesions and lower motor neuron lesions which is made in adults is not necessarily applicable to hypotonia in childhood.[265] In adults hypotonia would reflect a disease of the lower motor neuron but in childhood, hypotonia may be a symptom of upper (brain) or lower (spinal cord) motor neuron disease. Children who have developmental disabilities may manifest the symptom of hypotonia. Their hypotonia is usually due to diseases of the brain or to the secondary effect of systemic illness. The differential diagnosis of the symptom of hypotonia is broad. When confronted with a child who has hypotonia it is best to first determine which area in his neuromuscular axis is involved and then to determine the specific etiology.[266] For this reason the diseases commonly causing hypotonia in childhood have been divided into categories based on the anatomy of the neuromuscular system. These diseases will be discussed in the categories outlined in Table X.

The assessment of a child with hypotonia begins with a detailed history to determine if there are any associated factors in the family, if there are any important factors in the child's gestational history and life story, what the details are of the onset of the hypotonia and what other factors to which the child has been exposed. A careful general physical examination and a detailed neurological examination with particular attention paid to the motor system (Chapter 2) can give one an impression as to which categories are likely. A brief developmental evaluation (Chapter 2) will be helpful to decide whether the patient falls into the category of brain dysfunction.

From the data obtained in the history, the physical, neurolog

115

Table X

DIFFERENTIAL DIAGNOSIS OF HYPOTONIA IN INFANCY AND CHILDHOOD

I. Brain.
   A. Hypotonia of cerebral palsy.
   B. Storage and degenerative diseases of the CNS, e.g. Tay-Sachs.
   C. Aminoacidopathies.
   D. Chromosomal and genetic disorders, e.g. mongolism.
   E. Other encephalopathies, e.g. kernicterus.
II. Motor neuron (Anterior horn cell).
   A. Wernig-Hoffman disease (Infantile progressive muscular atrophy).
   B. Kügelberg-Welander disease (Hereditary juvenile muscular atrophy).
   C. Poliomyelitis.
   D. Myelopathic arthrogryposis multiplex congenita.
III. Nerve root or peripheral nerve.
   A. Landry-Guillain-Barré syndrome.
   B. Polyneuritis.
   C. Charcot-Marie-Tooth disease.
   D. Other
      1. Traumatic.
      2. Infectious.
      3. Toxic.
IV. Myoneural junction.
   A. Myasthenia gravis.
      1. Neonatal (transient).
      2. Congenital.
      3. Juvenile.
      4. Ocular.
   B. Other.
      1. Toxins of *Clostridium botulinum.*
      2. Venoms of cobra and arachnoideae.
V. Muscle.
   A. Muscular dystrophies.
      1. Congenital infantile muscular dystrophy with or without arthrogryposis.
      2. Duchenne's dystrophy.
      3. Facioscapulohumoral dystrophy.
      4. Limb-girdle dystrophy.
   B. Myotonic disorders.
      1. Myotonic dystrophy.
      2. Myotonia congenita.
      3. Paramyotonia congenita.
   C. Inflammatory muscle diseases.
      1. Dematomyositis.
      2. Polymyositis.
      3. Other.
         a. Viral infections.
         b. Collagen disease.
         c. Rheumatic fever.
         d. Rheumatoid arthritis.
         e. Trichinosis.
      4. Microscopic myopathies.
         a. Nemaline myopathy (rod body myopathy).
         b. Central core disease.
         c. Myotubular (centrotubular) myopathy.
         d. Myopathies with abnormal mitochondria.

5. Biochemical defects of muscle.
   a. Hypokalemic periodic paralysis.
   b. Hyperkalemic periodic paralysis.
   c. Muscle phosphoralase deficiency.
   d. Pompe's disease (Glycogen storage disease, Type II).
   e. Congenital defect of phosphofructokinase.
   f. Myoglobinuria.
VI. Benign congenital hypotonia.
VII. Other.
   A. Secondary effect of chronic diseases, e.g. congenital heart disease.
   B. Secondary effect of metabolic disorders, e.g. hypothyroidism.
   C. Emotional deprivation.

---

ical and developmental examinations, one could determine which specialized laboratory studies are needed to further delineate the etiology of the hypotonia. If one is questioning disease processes involving the motor unit, motor neurons, peripheral nerves or muscle, specialized studies of muscle enzymes (CPK and aldolase) may be helpful.[267] These enzymes are often elevated in processes where there is active muscle destruction, either primarily or secondarily. An EMG (electromyogram) and a NCV (nerve conduction velocity study) may be useful in the diagnostic evaluation of diseases of the muscle, the myoneural junction, the nerve, or the anterior horn cell.[268] In some instances, it may be necessary to perform a muscle biopsy. This may be diagnostic of primary muscle disease or anterior horn cell disease. There are some very specialized microscopic disease processes of muscle that can lead to hypotonia and it may be necessary to do special stains on frozen muscle biopsy specimens or electron microscopic examination of the specimen.[269]

Brain

Many of the disease processes in this category (see Table X) are discussed elsewhere in this text. One significant factor in this category is that in many of these disease processes, e.g. kernicterus, one expects to find hypertonia.[270, 271] However, there may be a transient period of hypotonia prior to the development of increased tone (spasticity), which is more characteristic of these conditions. Hypotonia may be a manifestation of cerebral palsy (Chapter 7).

Anterior Horn Cell

The anterior horn cell in the spinal cord is the lower motor neuron of the neuromuscular axis. The motor neurons in the brain stem that supply the cranial nerves (the nerves that supply the muscles of the head and neck) are embryologic analogs (Chapter 3) of the lower motor neuron cells of the anterior horn in the spinal cord. Therefore, disease processes that affect anterior horn cells also affect the neurons of the motor cranial nerve nuclei.

Today, the most commonly encountered disease process involving anterior horn cells is *Wernig-Hoffman's disease* (progressive infantile atrophy).[272] This disease process is inherited as an autosomal recessive condition. For reasons that have not been delineated, the anterior horn cells in Wernig-Hoffman's disease undergo changes, become atrophic, and die. The primary symptom of this disease is hypotonia. Wernig-Hoffman's disease may present at different ages during infancy. The earlier the appearance of Wernig-Hoffman's disease, the more fulminating its course and the more rapid the patient's downhill progression and death. For purposes of prognosis, Wernig-Hoffman has been divided into types according to age of onset.[273] Type I will have their symptoms manifested in the first two months of life, Type II between two and twelve months, and Type III between twelve and twenty-four months.

In Type I the mother may state that the child had decreased movements when it was in utero. Infants with Type I Wernig-Hoffman's disease will have very little movement of the muscles of the body except for the distal muscles of their hands and their feet. There may be involvement of the muscles of the chest wall and there may be even involvement of the diaphragm, further compromising their breathing capacity. The muscles of the cranial nerves are involved with Type I Wernig-Hoffman's disease so that the infant will have difficulty crying, swallowing, and sucking. These infants have difficulty handling their secretions and it is not infrequent that they succumb to aspiration pneumonia. These children never sit and never stand or walk. They may have absent deep tendon reflexes from birth. These children usually succumb to a complication of their illness by the age of two or three years.

Wernig-Hoffman Type II children may sit and may begin to stand, but as their disease progresses they lose these motor milestones and their motor development regresses. Their non-motor development proceeds at a normal rate so that speaking would occur at the expected age (see Chapter 1). These children have weakness usually of the proximal muscles of their arms and legs. The deep tendon reflex at the knee is usually the first reflex to disappear, but as the disease progresses they will lose all of their deep tendon reflexes. Although most of these children usually succumb to complications of their illness in the first decade of life, there are some Type II children who have a much slower course and they live to their teenage years.

Wernig-Hoffman Type III children do sit, stand, and may even walk. But, they lose their motor milestones as their disease progresses. When they present they usually show weakness at the thigh and hip. Very early in their disease they may have all the deep tendon reflexes, but their knee jerk is the first deep tendon reflex to be lost. As the disease progresses, they lose all of their deep tendon reflexes. Their nonmotor development proceeds at a normal rate. This disease does progress so that most children afflicted with Type III are confined to a wheelchair by their teenage years with death usually occurring in the late second or third decade.

The distinction between Wernig-Hoffman's disease and *Kügelberg-Welander's disease* (hereditary juvenile muscular atrophy) is based primarily on the age of onset of the condition since Kügelberg-Welander has its appearance between twenty-four months and seventeen years of age.[274] This disease process has the same neuropathology as Wernig-Hoffman. It is a disease process with progressive loss of anterior horn cells in the spinal cord. Kügelberg-Welander is an autosomal recessive condition with some autosomal dominant pedigrees. Patients with Kügelberg-Welander present with weakness in their legs and gait difficulties. Their hip and thigh muscles are affected first and they may initially show difficulty climbing up or down stairs. Weakness in the arms develops later than weakness in the legs. The first deep tendon reflex to disappear is the knee jerk, but as the disease progresses all deep tendon reflexes are lost. As the disease progresses muscular atrophy occurs and the patient loses the ability to ambulate. At least half of the persons afflicted with this disease live beyond twenty years of age and many individuals may live into their thirties and forties before succumbing to complications.

A definitive diagnosis of Wernig-Hoffman and Kügelberg-Welander can be made with muscle biopsy.[269] There is a very characteristic pattern on muscle biopsy with groups of muscle fibers supplied by these same anterior horn cells showing atrophy adjacent to groups of muscle fibers supplied by nondefective anterior horn cells appearing normal. This pattern is referred to as grouped atrophy. The electromyogram may give some clues to this diagnosis because muscles that are being denervated by their anterior horn cell may have spontaneous activity and these signs of spontaneous activity (fibrillations) may be detected on the electromyogram. At times, evidence of denervation can be seen by observing the patient for muscle fasciculations or involuntary muscle twitching. These can be seen through the skin of patients who are thin. It is not unusual for normal individuals occasionally to experience muscle fasciculations. In normal individuals, these are benign sporadic fasciculations in contrast to the persistent frequent fasciculations seen in the Wernig-Hoffman and Kügelberg-Welander disease. Muscle enzymes (CPK and aldolase) may be normal or only slightly elevated in these disease processes.[267]

Poliomyelitis is now a relatively infrequent cause of anterior horn cell disease in childhood. Polio belongs to the group of viruses called enterovirus. The polio virus in particular has the propensity to attack the nervous system in man and specifically attack the motor neurons in the nervous system.[276] The neurons primarily involved are the anterior horn cell neurons and the motor cranial nerve neurons. It is important to realize that any of the enterovirus are capable of producing selective disease of the anterior horn cells and motor nuclei of the nervous system. The coxachie virus or echo virus may produce a picture quite like polio.[277] Although the patient has been immunized against polio, it is possible that other enteroviral types may attack the nervous system in a similar fashion to the polio virus, producing the same clinical picture.

Arthrogryposis multiplex congenita is a descriptive term. It defines a condition where there are multiple flexion contractures of joints present at the time of birth.[278] It is possible to have arthrogryposis multiplex congenita on the basis of pathology of the brain or of the spinal cord (myelopathic) or in the nerves (neuropathic) or in the joints or in the muscle (myopathic). Should one be fortunate enough to relieve these contractures with physical therapy the underlying muscles will be found to be hypotonic.[279]

Nerve Root or Peripheral Nerve

The *Landry-Guillain-Barré syndrome* is felt to be a secondary sequela of a viral illness.[280] It is thought to be an autoimmune process that arises after exposure to certain viral agents. In the classical form, it is characterized by an ascending muscular paralysis beginning in the ankles and gradually ascending. In some instances individuals may have paralysis of the respiratory muscles and will require a respirator. It is important to diagnose this condition and treat it promptly since individuals who paralyze their muscles of respiration may expire. Individuals who are afflicted with Landry-Guillain-Barré syndrome have an elevation in their spinal fluid protein. They may have involvement of sensory as well as motor function. Treatment for this condition is supportive with 80 percent of the cases in childhood being completely reversible.[281]

Polyneuropathies are uncommon in childhood. They may occur secondary to certain toxins, but these conditions are rarely seen in childhood. In polyneuropathies there is temporary or permanent demyelination of peripheral nerves so that they do not function normally. The clinical manifestation of motor neuropathy is weakness in an area.[282] Depending on the etiology, there may be sensory involvement as well. There is usually an elevation of their spinal fluid protein and nerve conduction velocities become slowed as the disease progresses.

Charcot-Marie-Tooth is a familial condition that is usually inherited as an autosomal dominant fashion. These individuals will have progressive weakness of the muscles in their feet and calves and gradually have involvement in muscles of their thighs. Frequently, there is some cerebellar involvement and there are some noscologists who would classify this condition with other genetic spinal cerebellar degenerations.[283]

Myoneural Junction

Myasthenia gravis is a chronic disease characterized by unusual fatiguability of muscle. There are several different clinical presentations of this disease, which include a neonatal (transient) form, a congenital form, a juvenile form, and an ocular form.[284] Neonatal transient myasthenia gravis occurs in one out of seven infants born to myasthenic mothers.[285] The symptoms usually appear in the first twenty-four hours of life but clearly appear by the third day of life. Symptoms usually last up to five weeks, but in some instances they may persist for several months. In all instances, there is weakness of the lower bulbar muscles causing a weak cry, difficulty swallowing, and difficulty sucking. Fifty percent of patients will have generalized hypotonia. It is important to diagnose this condition, because it is treatable with anticholinesterase medications and is reversible. Children with transient myasthenia gravis will effect a full recovery since they merely reflect a disease process in the mother.

In congenital myasthenia gravis, the infants are born to mothers who do not have myasthenia gravis.[286] The symptoms are persistent throughout life. Mothers of congenital myasthenic children may have noted decreased fetal movements during gestation. These infants usually have feeding difficulties and weak cries during the newborn period. They may also have ptosis, facial weakness, and diffuse weakness. Their symptom of weakness may vary like adult myasthenic patients.

Juvenile myasthenia presents in the age bracket of two years through adolescence.[286] Its onset may be rapid or insidious. Oftentimes it seems to follow a febrile or viral illness. The clinical course of this condition is variable. In severe cases, weakness may spread to the respiratory muscles and produce death within a few months despite treatment. Most patients will experience a remission early in their illness and be troubled with the symptoms that wax and wane. Ocular myasthenia occurs in about 5 percent of the cases of myasthenia gravis. This form of myasthenia is restricted to the ocular muscles. Treatment is usually unsatisfactory and the patient will report impairment of vision, double vision or ptosis of the eyelids as they fatigue.

In general, myasthenic patients have variations in their muscle strength. The child is usually at his best in the morning and becomes weaker as the day progresses, getting better after he rests. In 10 to 20 percent of the patients, weakness may become irreversible and generalized muscle wasting particularly around the shoulders may become apparent. Despite the hypotonia in these individuals, the deep tendon reflexes may be increased or normal. With juvenile myasthenia, thyroid disease occurs in approximately 10 percent of the individuals.

The diagnosis of myasthenia gravis is often difficult since the patient has weakness that comes and goes. The disease itself is subject to periods of remission. The individual will often feel better and normally strong at certain points during the day, but his muscles will fatigue as they are used. For example, individuals who have involvement about their fingers complain of weakness or possibly stiffness of their muscles after doing repetitive acts such as knitting.

The diagnosis of myasthenia can be made often with medications.[287] The medications used for testing are edrophonium chloride (Tensilon®) or neostigmine. The symptom of weakness would dissipate following the administration of the medication, but the result is only transient. A specialized EMG with repetitive stimulation may show the muscles to fatigue easily under stress. Occasionally, a muscle biopsy may show some infiltration of inflammatory cells (lymphoid series) around muscle fibers.

Patients with myasthenia will respond to treatment with anticholinesterase agents and/or steroids. The lesion in myasthenia gravis is at the myoneural junction (the synapse between the nerve and the muscle) where acetylcholine (the transmitter substance which stimulates muscle movement) is liberated.

The *toxins* liberated by certain bacteria particularly *Clostridium botulinum*, venoms from certain snakes and spiders and organophosphates are capable of producing transient blockage at the neuromuscular junction.[288, 289] One condition, infantile botulism, has received significant attention recently.[290] This condition, which affects infants in the first few months of life, is manifested by a gradual onset of weakness. Weakness progresses to paralysis that may involve the muscles of respiration. In infantile botulism, the toxin of *Clostridium botulinum* cannot be appreciated in the blood stream, but the spores of the organism can be seen in the gastrointestinal tract. It is important to diagnose this condition since it is completely reversible. Treatment consists of supportive care and ventilatory assistance if necessary.

Muscle

Some children are born with *congenital muscular dystrophy*.[291, 292] This is a hereditary disease in which the child may manifest myopathic arthrogryposis multiplex congenita. There is a type of congenital muscular dystrophy with universal hypoplasia (smallness) of the muscle fibers. This is a nonprogressive condition in contrast to most other forms of muscular dystrophy.

The following are the common forms of muscular dystrophy: Duchenne's dystrophy, facioscapulohumoral dystrophy, and limb-girdle dystrophy.[264, 293] There are a group of hereditary disease with gradual onset of weakness. There is a loss of deep tendon reflexes as the disease progresses. There may be atrophy of muscle groups, but in some conditions there may be pseudohypertrophy of muscles.

The most common dystrophy of childhood is *Duchenne's muscular dystrophy*. This is a sex-linked recessive condition that, by definition, affects only males. There have been a few unusual instances of females with Duchenne's dystrophy reported. The onset of the illness is in early childhood, usually presenting by six years of age. Since its onset is gradual, the early symptoms may be overlooked. Early symptoms may include clumsiness, difficulty climbing stairs, or difficulty arising from the floor. Curvatures of the spine (scoliosis) may become apparent. As the disease progresses, the patient may show a waddling gait since the pelvic girdle muscles are usually affected first. Over 80 percent of individuals affected with Duchenne's dystrophy show pseudohypertrophy of their muscles at some point in the disease. Most children afflicted with Duchenne's dystrophy have a rapid progression of weakness, loss of motor function and death due to intercurrent infections in the second or third decades.

Generally, there is a diminution of intellectual capacity in these children. Their intelligence quotients are usually in the borderline or low-normal range. There is a small group of individuals (approximately 10 percent) with Duchenne's dystrophy who have a very slowly progressive form of the disease with a later age of onset. In approximately 50 to 80 percent of individuals, the heart muscles will become involved and cardiac failure may occur. In the early phase of this condition, the serum muscle enzymes (CPK and aldolase) are markedly elevated. The EMG shows a very characteristic pattern of muscle disease. The muscle biopsy can be confirmatory in Duchenne's and other muscular dystrophies, showing variation in muscle fiber size.

Facioscapulohumoral dystrophy is a form of muscular dystrophy that affects the muscles about the face, the shoulders, and the upper arms. It is usually an autosomal dominant condition. There may be a great variation in the clinical course of individuals affected with facioscapulohumoral dystrophy. In general, the clinical course of a given pedigree is the same so that each affected family member will follow a similar clinical course. The initial symptoms are usually shoulder girdle weakness, prominent winging of the scapula, thinning of neck muscles and development of *myopathic facies* with lips that cannot be pursed and approximated. The myopathic face appears rather triangular with slightly protuberant lips. The age of onset varies from late childhood to early adult years. Pseudohypertrophy is uncommonly seen. Contractures and cardiac involvement are very rarely seen and intellectual capacity is normal.

Limb-girdle muscular dystrophy represents a broad group of clinical conditions. They are usually autosomal recessive but some dominant forms are seen. As in the facioscapulohumoral, pedigrees are consistent in their involvement. The weakness in limb-girdle dystrophy usually appears in the second or third decade of life and involves primarily the shoulder and/or pelvic girdles. Less than 30 percent will show pseudohypertrophy. The course of the disease and the rate of progression is highly variable according to the pedigree. Contractures may develop late in the disease. Cardiac involvement is exceptionally rare and intelligence is normal.

Myotonic Disorders

Muscle myotonia is defined as the failure of voluntary muscles to relax normally after contraction. Patients may complain of having difficulty letting go of objects. Clinically, the symptom of myotonia can be elicited by having the patient grasp and release an object and observing their slow relaxation response. Myotonia may be demonstrated by percussion of muscles with a reflex hammer and observing the muscle contract and then relax at a much slower rate than normal. Myotonia can be seen in many conditions.

The most common disease of muscle associated with myotonia is *myotonic dystrophy*.[294] This autosomal dominant condition may start early in life. The age of onset appears to become earlier with each subsequently afflicted generation. As the disease progresses, muscular atrophy, weakness, and myopathic facies begin to appear. Muscles about the sternocleidomastoid, the shoulder, and pelvic girdles begin to atrophy as the disease progresses. Mental retardation is seen in as high as 80 percent of individuals afflicted with myotonic dystrophy. About half of the patients will have some disturbance of cardiac function. Other symptoms associated with this condition include cataracts, endocrine disturbances with testicular atrophy, diabetes mellitus, frontal baldness, and loss of body hair. Late in its course, this disease may be associated with the development of dementia (a regression in intellectual performance). The diagnosis can be suspected by eliciting the positive family history, the symptom of myotonia, or the characteristic myopathic facies. The EMG can be exceptionally helpful in confirming the diagnosis since the inability of the muscle to relax after a single firing can be demonstrated on the EMG.

Myotonia is present in *myotonia congenita* (Thompson's disease). This disease presents as hypotonia in infancy. This is an autosomal dominant disease with many sporadic forms. It is a nonprogressive condition and individuals will have a normal lifespan.

Paramyotonia is a condition of a more benign nature where the mytonia is associated with exposure to cold. Individuals who have this difficulty will experience inability of their muscles to relax only during exposure to cold. Some individuals may also have attacks of generalized weakness associated with increases in serum potassium (see hyperkalemic periodic paralysis below).

Inflammatory Diseases of Muscle

Dematomyositis is a form of collagen vascular disease.[295] Individuals afflicted with this condition often have low grade fevers, easy fatiguability, anorexia, signs of generalized weakness, and muscle pain. They usually have an insidious onset but may have an acute onset precipitated by an infection. Often they have an associated skin rash manifested by a *violaceous discoloration* of the upper eyelids and the extensor surfaces of the joints particularly about the knuckles. Deep tendon reflexes in this condition are diminished or absent. The disease has a quite variable course, but up to 75 percent of patients afflicted will expire despite therapy. Diagnostic laboratory data includes an elevation in sedimentation rate and an electromyogram showing fibrillations and myopathic changes. A muscle biopsy will be diagnostic if it shows inflammatory cells around the muscle fibers. Treatment can be successful with corticosteroids.

Polymyositis is a disease of a similar nature to dematomyositis except that the cutaneous skin manifestations are not present.[296] Also, myositis may be seen with other collagen diseases, e.g. rheumatic fever and rheumatoid arthritis. A *benign myositis* may be seen secondary to viral illnesses. Myositis seen in these instances is usually transient, abating without therapy. Myositis may also be a manifestation of infection with the pork tapeworm that produces *trichinosis*.[297]

Microscopic Diseases of Muscle

There are several unusual and infrequently seen diseases of muscle where the diagnostic muscle defect can be appreciated on special anatomical studies of the muscle. These include diseases such as nemaline myopathy, central core disease, myotubular myopathy, and mitochondrial myopathy. In *nema-*

line myopathy, the disease is an autosomal dominant or occasionally a recessive condition that is present at birth.[298] It is a nonprogressive or slowly progressive condition. The hallmark of the condition is the finding of red colored particles on trichrome stain of the muscle at the time of biopsy.

Central core disease is an autosomal dominant condition that, like nemaline myopathy, may be present at birth, but is nonprogressive in nature.[299] Its diagnosis is made by trichrome stain. The muscle fibers in this disease will stain the central area with a blue color and the peripheral area with a red color indicating some distortion in the normal anatomy of the muscle fiber.

Myotubular (centrotubular) myopathy is a progressive condition with weakness of the limbs, girdle, and neck muscles.[300] Ptosis and weakness of the extraocular muscles may be seen. The hallmark of this condition pathologically is the presence of central or internal nuclei in the muscle fiber. Some investigators feel that this represents a developmental arrest in muscle maturation since the fibers appear much like the fibers of fetal muscles.

There are a series of diseases that show weakness secondary to some abnormalities of the muscle cell mitrochondria (subcellular organelles). The *mitochondrial myopathies* are diagnostic only by electron microscopic examination of muscle tissue.[301] They tend to be hereditofamilial diseases with variable pedigree specific prognoses.

Biochemical Defects of Muscle

Biochemical defects of intermittent or persistent nature may cause episodic paralysis or permanent paralysis of the muscle group. *Hypokalemic periodic paralysis* is an autosomal dominant condition that is characterized by intermittent acute transient muscle paralyses lasting for six to twenty-four hours. These episodes can be serious, with death occurring in 10 percent of attacks when there is paralysis of muscles of respiration. During an attack, there is a drop in muscle potassium, but it is transient. The serum must be sampled at the time of attack in order to make the diagnosis. Individuals afflicted with this condition develop progressive muscular atrophy.[302]

Hyperkalemic periodic paralysis is another autosomal dominant condition which will cause muscle paralysis.[303] Ninety percent of the cases have their onset before ten years of age. Attacks may occur up to one to two times a week and are usually precipitated by rest following physical exertion with each attack lasting approximately half an hour. The patient often complains of weakness in the muscles about the hip girdle. In many individuals with hyperkalemic periodic paralysis, a history of paramyotonia may be obtained and/or percussion myotonia may be seen. During an attack, there is an elevation in serum potassium and attacks can be precipitated by infusing the patient with potassium. Many patients experience relief from their attacks with azetazolamide (Chapter 6) therapy.

McArdle's disease is an autosomal recessive condition where there is a lack of the enzyme, muscle phosphoralase.[304] Attacks begin in early childhood with muscle cramps following exercise. Episodes of myoglobinuria (urine darkened by muscle breakdown products) may be seen with this condition. After exercise, the individuals with McArdle's disease are not able to eliminate lactic acid (a metabolite produced with muscle exercise) from their muscles. The muscle biopsy may be confirmatory in this condition if it shows an increase in glycogen. Another form of congenital muscle enzyme deficit is phosphofructokinase deficiency.[305] The clinical picture is very similar to McArdle's disease. The diagnosis can be made by doing a phosphofructokinase level assay in red blood cells.

There are a variety of conditions in which episodic myoglobinuria may occur as a reflection of muscle tissue destruction.[306] These are unusual conditions that tend to be genetic. The enzyme deficit(s) has (have) not been elucidated at this time, although muscle carnitine deficiency has been found in some cases.

Benign Congenital Hypotonia

Benign congenital hypotonia was first described by Walton in the 1950s.[307] It is a syndrome that is characterized by hypotonia being present from the time of birth, by a negative history of neuromuscular disease, negative evaluation of the neuromuscular system (including muscle enzymes, NCV, EMG and biopsy) and progressive improvement with age. Most children afflicted with benign congenital hypotonia have normal muscle strength and tone by the time they are 2 to 3 years of age.

Amyotonia congenita is a term that was popular in the literature until recently. This was taken to be a pathological entity when it was first described by Oppenheim in the early 1900s. He described a group of infants who were hypotonic at the time of birth and found that they either improved, got progressively worse or stayed the same. No pathological studies were performed on these patients.[308] Today we realize that a heterogeneous group of conditions was described. The ones who improved probably were benign congenital hypotonia. Those that worsened were most likely Wernig-Hoffman's disease or progressive myopathies. Those whose weakness stayed the same probably represented forms of congenital nonprogressive myopathies.

Other

Hypotonia may be seen as a manifestation of *severe deprivation in infancy*. This diagnosis can only be made after a negative complete neuromuscular evaluation. Signs of psychological and/or physical deprivation in the child may be present. Children who are afflicted with hypotonia as a result of deprivation will show a rapid improvement in their muscle tone following intensive substitute mothering programs.[309]

Hypotonia in infancy and childhood may be a secondary manifestation of any chronic disease. Diseases that may produce hypotonia include congenital heart disease and severe malnutrition. In these conditions, the hypotonia will become corrected when the primary disease process is ameliorated. Hypotonia may be a reflection of nervous system dysfunction seen in systemic diseases such as hypothyroidism, or chromosomal and genetic diseases such as Down's syndrome where the hypotonia is part of the central nervous system dysfunction.

Chapter 9

AUTISM

$\mathbf{A}$UTISM IS A descriptive term for the tendency toward self absorption with an inanimate regard for or fear of human beings. Leo Kanner described a specific form of autism that he called infantile autism.[310] Infantile autism is a severe emotional disturbance of infancy and early childhood. It is characterized by an inability of the infant or child to relate with people in a meaningful way. After Kanner's description of infantile autism there was a great tendency to consider all infants and children who manifested autistic behavior as part of the symptom complex of infantile autism. In actuality, autism or autistic behavior is really a descriptive term rather than a diagnostic entity. When a child is diagnosed as having autistic behavior it is important to ascertain the etiology of the autistic behavior since the treatment will vary according to its etiology. Causes of autistic behavior (see Table XI) include true infantile autism, autistic behavior secondary to neurological factors, and autistic behavior secondary to psychosocial factors.[310-314]

In earlier chapters, we have emphasized the influence of neurotoxic agents on neurological function and developmental progress in affected individuals. Just as areas of the brain that control motor function, reading function and sensory function can be damaged, areas that control behavioral functions may also be damaged by neurotoxic agents.[311] It is quite possible that aberrant behavioral patterns that would have the symptoms of autistic behavior may result from neurotoxic insults. Individuals manifesting this dysfunction may or may not show other signs of neurological dysfunction, such as soft neurological signs, developmental delays, spasticity, or seizure disorders.

There are several forms of storage and degenerative diseases (Appendix B) whose earliest manifestations may be behavioral changes or whose progressive neurodysfunctional changes may include behavioral abnormalities. The children afflicted with

Table XI

DIFFERENTIAL DIAGNOSIS OF AUTISM

    I. Primary — true infantile autism.
   II. Secondary.
        A. Neurological.
            1. Postneurotoxic insult.
            2. Progressive storage or degenerative disease.
            3. Sensory organ damage.
        B. Psychosocial.
            1. Infantile or childhood schizophrenia.
            2. Maternal-child symbiosis.
            3. Deprivation.

these difficulties may show autistic behavior as part of their symptom complex. Children who are deprived of normal sensory stimuli, such as deaf children, may appear to be living in a world of their own with a morbid self absorption. Their symptom of autism may merely be a reflection of their lack of sensory stimuli.

Infants and children are somewhat limited in their capacity to respond to psychosocial stress. One way for him to respond to such stress is to withdraw and become morbidly preoccupied with himself to the exclusion of other human beings in his environment.[316] This is seen as a symptom in childhood schizophrenia whether it be endogenous or secondary to a psychotraumatic event.[314] This behavior of morbid self absorption may also be seen in maternal child symbiosis when the mother is not present in the child's environment. Severe emotional deprivation or severe environmental deprivation may lead to the symptom of morbid self absorption and fear of or inanimate regard of other human beings.

Many of the characteristics of true infantile autism as described by Leo Kanner are seen in children with secondary autistic behavior. Although it is often difficult to separate the individual types, several factors are seemingly important: (1) The child with true infantile autism will have had autistic behavior from the time of birth; (2) there will be no history of neurotoxic insults pre- or postnatally; (3) the child's formal neurological examination is normal; and (4) there is no history of psychotraumatic events.

True infantile autism as described by Leo Kanner refers to children who have a disturbance of affect. These children's outstanding feature was an inability to relate to human beings in an ordinary way. Loretta Bender further defined infantile autism on the basis of primary and secondary factors.[317] Primary factors included the following: (1) extreme autistic aloneness; and (2) an anxious obsessive desire to preserve sameness in the environment, daily routine or experience. Secondary factors included the following: (1) a skillful relationship with nonhuman objects; (2) an intelligent appearing child who had some isolated areas of high competency; (3) low level of intellectual performance on formalized testing; and (4) a language disturbance. The language disturbance in these children would include complete mutism, noncommunicative language, bizarre language disturbance, or simply the failure of usage of the first person pronoun.

The extreme autistic aloneness of these children is present from the early start of their life. Close questioning of parents may reveal that this was present from the very beginning of life. The average child at the age of four months will make anticipatory motor adjustments by altering his facial tension with a shrugging attitude of the shoulders when parents come by to lift him from his crib.[3] True infantile autistic children never assumed the anticipatory posture prior to being picked up. Parents will often say these children are happiest when they are left alone. Whenever possible, the child ignores, disregards, and tries to shut out anything in the environment that is outside himself. It is this extreme tendency for aloneness with absorption into self that is present from the very beginning of life that differentiates true infantile autism from the childhood psychosis and from deprived children.

Children with infantile autism dread change. They are content doing a monotonous repetitive task with limitation in variety and limitation in spontaneous activity. These monotonous repetitious tasks are of their own choosing. In addition, they have an anxious obsessive desire to maintain their order and sameness in their environment and to maintain a consistent daily routine that only the child may disrupt on occasion.

Children with infantile autism regard inanimate objects and human beings both in a similar manner. They do not make eye contact with humans. Their approach to a human is the same as their approach to an inanimate object.[318] They prefer objects to humans because of the former's consistency in appearance and position in contrast to humans who change their expression and their position.

It is difficult to adequately assess the intelligence of a child with true infantile autism. Since these children appear normally bright and alert and they can excel in certain tasks on developmental testing, many people assume that their underlying intelligence is normal.[319] However, when given a formal battery of intellectual tests they will succeed well only in certain areas and have an overall depressed intellectual quotient.[320] It is not unusual for an infantile autistic child to be labeled as retarded or deaf because of their inability to perform on developmental or audiometric testing.

The language disturbance in infantile autism is variable.[321] In the original eleven patients described by Leo Kanner, three were mute and eight spoke at the usual age but with some delay in the cadence of speech development (Chapter 1). These individuals were capable of speech but their language may have been of their own jargon. They may have an excellent memory and may be able to repeat nursery rhymes, prayers, poems, or songs at an early age, but will do little else with language.

Many of these children will have a delayed echolalia where they will repeat word combinations at later times. Often personal pronouns are misused. They appear not to be able to distinguish the *I*'s from the *you*'s from the *its* and *we*'s. Many times their speech takes on a rather concrete pattern. For example, a father who wanted his child to say *please* would say "If you want me to pick you up and put you on my shoulders, say please." To this child with infantile autism, the word *please* may mean pick me up and put me on your shoulders. A mother might say to an autistic child "Now I will pour your milk" and this child when he wants milk would repeat "Now I will pour your milk."

Kanner made some observations concerning the family units from which children with infantile autism were descended. He found that the children came from highly intelligent families with many nationally acclaimed individuals in science, literature and the arts. He felt that many of the marriages were unsuccessful and cold and that the parents were professional and emotionally undemonstrable people. However, it appears that he was dealing with a highly selected group who sought out his services and these observations concerning family structure are no longer applicable.

After Kanner's description of infantile autism, many individuals attempted to determine the etiology of this condition. Benda felt that autism was a result of a diffuse encephalopathy.[317] Later, Kanner proposed that emotional isolation and obsessiveness were etiologic.[322] Bettelheim felt the disorder to be primarily psychogenic.[319] Rutter felt that there was a basic defect in the comprehension and appreciation of sound.[311] Rimland postulated that these children suffered hypoxia at birth causing undemonstrable lesions in the reticular formation of the brain.[323]

All of these investigators were describing etiological factors responsible for producing autistic behavior in some individuals (see Table XI). It is now apparent that autistic behavior is merely a symptom and not a synonym for the original infantile autism described by Leo Kanner. In order to initiate appropriate treatment, it is important to determine which form of autistic behavior is present in a given child. This detailed evaluation would involve at least a neurologist, psychologist, psychiatrist, pediatrician, and social worker for a complete assessment to be undertaken. It is unusually best handled by an interdisciplinary team.

Historical information is important in the assessment of the child's early neurological and psychosocial development. When the child responded with a smile to a familiar face is an important historical factor. The average child does this by four to six weeks of age.[3] This information may give one a clue as to how a mother felt about the child from early in his infancy or as to how the child responded to her. For example, a mother who says her child never smiles, but always cries may have had early negative feelings toward the child. Whereas the mother who said that the child smiled whenever she came in his presence from four weeks on probably had an appropriate early relationship with the child.

Another landmark of importance is whether the child made anticipatory motor and/or postural movements and adjustments in facial tension when the parent approached the child in his crib. Normally children from four to six months of age will make anticipatory postures to a parent when he desires to be picked up.[3] Autistic children fail to communicate at any age and therefore would not show any anticipatory postures when approached.

A detailed history of motor and speech development is important since in children with true infantile autism the motor development usually is normal but speech development is usually abnormal. Although they may begin uttering the repetitive syllables at the appropriate age (six to none months), their speech may fail to progress at a normal rate. A child with a global developmental lag may have a delay in his motor milestones and also a delay in the cadence of speech development with repetitive syllables and whole words developing at later than normal (Chapter 1). The quality of speech is important as well, e.g. the child's ability to repeat word combinations; the child's ability to memorize nursery rhymes, poems, songs and prayers.[321]

A detailed review of the gestational and perinatal history of the child should be undertaken looking for signs of possible neurotoxic insults. A general physical examination looking for any stigmata of diseases associated with developmental disabilities (Appendix C) is important. A detailed formal neurological examination (Chapter 2) that would be looking toward any associated defects such as evidence of motor dysfunction or cranial nerve palsies would be important. It is also important to repeat neurological examination at given periods in time looking for the appearance of new neurological deficits that would point toward a regressive disease, such as degenerative or storage disease (Appendix B). A detailed developmental examination is exceptionally useful. This should be done by one who is very skilled in performing developmental testing. Particular attention should be paid to the child's overall performance and his performance on various subtests. In general, children with true infantile autism perform better on nonverbal rather than verbal testing.

In addition, specialized tests such as speech and hearing evaluations would be important to determine if the child is capable of hearing. Brain stem auditory evoked response would be useful because it is an electrical test that can determine if sound is being picked up by the child's brain stem requiring no cooperation from the child.[324] Many autistic children do not respond in the normal way to speech.

An EEG is a useful test to assess a child with autistic behavior looking for signs of cerebral dysfunction. There is one form of autistic behavior secondary to neurological insult where there will be a spike focus in the temporal recording areas.[326] These children's behavior is often helped by treatment with an anticonvulsant medication such as phenytoin. In addition, computerized axial tomographic study of the brain would be important looking for gross anatomical defects within the nervous system.[159]

A psychiatric evaluation of the child and his family as well as a detailed psychiatric history would be important to determine if there were any negative parental attitudes toward the child, any signs of deprivation, or any psychotraumatic events that occurred during the child's life that may have precipitated the behavioral abnormality. A child with autistic behavior secondary to psychosocial trauma will have had normal function until the traumatic event.

The treatment for autistic behavior varies according to etiology.[311, 327] For children with true infantile autism, the best treatment available is intensive one-to-one therapy. In this therapy, the therapist attempts initially to form eye contact; later, an interpersonal relationship is formed with the child, and, finally, this relationship is transferred to other individuals. Even with intensive therapy, which usually requires day or permanent institutional care, the prognosis for infantile autism is somewhat guarded. It can be anticipated however that approximately 50 percent will have good usage language and approximately 30 to 40 percent will be able to function normally in society.[310, 312, 315] One of the critical factors that influences the prognosis in infantile autism is the time therapy was initiated. The earlier the therapy is initiated the better the prognosis.

For individuals who have autistic behavior secondary to childhood psychosis, intensive therapy involving the child and/or the family may improve the prognosis. In addition, anti-psychotic medication may be useful adjuncts to treatment. For individuals with deprivation, the child needs to be removed from his depriving environment and, through proper regressive techniques, intensive substitute mothering techniques,[308] and therapy for the parents, the child may become normally functional.

The prognosis for children with autistic behavior secondary to neurological damage is guarded.[311] If there is sensory organ damage, attempts at compensation for the sensory deprivation through the functional organ systems can be instituted, or, if possible, repair of the damaged sensory organ. Children with neurogenic or neurotoxic insults usually are not responsive to intensive forms of therapy and often are better served with behavior modification techniques. Medical therapy should be instituted whenever necessary. Children with degenerative or neuronal storage diseases have poor prognosis for life. In many instances, children with neurogenic causes of autistic behavior also have some psychosocial deprivation to compound their problems so that intensive substitute mothering techniques may be beneficial for these children as well.[309]

Summary

Autism is a term that describes a peculiar behavior in which the infant or child prefers to be alone with a morbid self absorption. His relationship with humans is comparable to that with inanimate objects. Autistic behavior is merely a symptom, and, in order for appropriate treatment to be undertaken, it is imperative that the etiology of the autistic behavior be determined since not all autistic behavior is a manifestation of true infantile autism.

Chapter 10

HYPERACTIVITY

HYPERACTIVITY can be defined as excessive motor activity for age. Associated with this is an inability to concentrate on the task at hand. Hyperactivity may be constant or it may be intermittent. Hyperactivity is not a diagnostic term but a descriptive term. It is a symptom, and, as any other symptom, it has multiple etiologies. Therefore, the treatment of hyperactivity depends upon the etiology of the symptom. Although there are numerous schemas that attempt to quantitate hyperactivity, there is no uniformly accepted scheme to accurately quantitate the severity of this complaint.[328-334] This may relate to the variability of some individual's symptoms with environmental or endogenous factors.

Like any other symptom complexes, there are multiple treatments depending on etiology. Unfortunately, the symptom of hyperactivity has a very high placebo response to any form of treatment. Placebo effect is seen in as much as 30 to 40 percent of cases.[335] The high placebo effect could be the failure of investigators to separate out different types of hyperactivity. The difficulty is quantitating the symptom has contributed to our poor understanding of this complaint. A basic framework is required before we can discuss hyperactivity since all children who manifest the symptom of overactivity do not represent one diagnostic category. Hyperactive children can be separated into two basic categories (see Table XII): constitutional (primary) and hyperactivity that is secondary to another problem. Children with constitutional hyperactivity have an innate inability to control their activity level. Children with secondary hyperactivity manifest the symptom in response to another basic problem.[336]

A multidisciplinary team approach is usually necessary to accurately evaluate the child with the complaint of hyperactivity. In addition to assessment of the history of the hyperactivity, it is important to take a detailed gestational history, a neurodevelop-

Table XII
DIFFERENTIAL DIAGNOSIS OF HYPERACTIVITY

I. Constitutional (Primary).
II. Secondary.
    A. Neurological (Organic).
        1. Associated with soft neurological signs and/or mild developmental disabilities.
        2. Associated with hard neurological signs and/or moderate to severe developmental disabilities.
    B. Psychosocial.
        1. Associated with emotional deprivation.
        2. Associated with situational stress.
        3. Associated with childhood neurosis.
        4. Associated with childhood psychosis/aggressiveness.
    C. Other.

---

mental history, a social and developmental history, family history, school history, and past medical history. A general physical examination is required as is a detailed neurological examination looking for soft neurological signs as well as gross neurological deficits. A developmental evaluation is important and a specialized evaluation of vision or hearing may be necessary. Evaluation of the family or home situation or the school situation may also be necessary. There is no place for an electroencephalographic evaluation. Before successful treatment of the hyperactivity can be instituted, a detailed evaluation to determine the cause should be undertaken.

The remainder of this chapter will be devoted to a discussion of the different forms of hyperactivity and the specific treatment for each type (see Table X).

Constitutional Hyperactivity

Children with primary hyperactivity have one or more of the following traits: (1) They have a very high energy level and expend a great amount of energy over the twenty-four-hour period of a day with much of their energy going into motor movements. (2) They have an inefficient regulatory control of their motor impulse. They may have much excessive movement, and, because their movements are excessive and quick, they may appear to be uncoordinated. Because of their misdirected overproduction of motor energy, they may find it difficult to perform fine motor tasks. (3) They have perpetual distractability. This may relate to a difficulty focusing their attention on the task at hand. These children begin to focus on an individual task, but are distracted easily by any irrelevant stimuli.[336]

As infants they may have been colicky. In general they slept little. They never played with any one object for long periods of time. As toddlers they never really walked but got up and ran. Their motor milestones are usually normal or accelerated for their developmental age. Often they will wake up at night, not because they are frightened or ill, but because they want to get up and get busy. As infants and young children they tend not to want to be cuddled but want to get going and get into many different things. They may be fearless and rather oblivious to danger. These children may have multiple accidents and injuries and may get into poisons.

Although these children are generally happy when they are young, later in life they may begin to have interactional difficulties at home or at school. In school, they get into difficulty because of their inability to focus in on the task at hand and by their ability to be easily distracted by extraneous stimuli. As older children they can get into difficulty because of complaints of forgetfulness and irresponsibility. When these children go to do a given task, they become distracted by external stimuli and drift off into something else, leaving the chore that they intended to accomplish unattended and incomplete.

Often, these children present between two and three years of age from middle or upper class families. They often present at school age from the lower socioeconomic groups when they are picked up by the teacher. An essential feature in these children is their impulsive approach to new situations or events and their inability to control their impulsiveness. These children are unable to attend to situations consistently. Threats and punishments are ineffective. Behavior modification is not helpful, but may drive the child and his family into a spiraling frenzy of frustration.

Children with primary hyperactivity may actually represent a lag in acquiring the normal control for attention control.[337] Hence, the term *developmental hyperactivity* has been applied to this group of children. Children with constitutional hyperactivity have no soft or hard neurological signs or deficits and no psychosocial deficits.

Individuals who use the term *developmental hyperactivity* would include in that group not only children with constitutional (primary) hyperactivity, but also children with neurogenic hyperactivity with soft neurological signs or minimal developmental disabilities. This group of children (constitutional and neurogenic with soft signs) would comply with the newly coined term *attention deficit disorder*.[338, 339]

Most children with constitutional hyperactivity *eventually* will be able to control their activity level regardless of whether treatment is instituted. However, in order to prevent the secondary interactional difficulties that may occur with these children as well as the poor school performance, it is wise to treat these children. Children with constitutional hyperactivity usually respond to stimulant medication.[340] Although it was initially thought that stimulant medication acted in a paradoxical manner with children who are hyperactive, current thinking favors the theory of these children responding in a manner similar to adults. They are stimulated by the medication so that they are then able to concentrate on one task and not be distracted by extraneous events.[341, 342]

The two most commonly used stimulant medications are methylphenidate (Ritalin®) and dextroamphetamine.[343] The dosage of methylphenidate can be calculated whether on the basis of body weight (0.2 to 0.4 mg/kg/24 hours) or by starting at a low dose and titrating the child's symptoms with response to medication.[344, 345] The starting dosage of methylphenidate would be 5 to 10 mg twice a day depending on the child's age. The usual starting dose of dextroamphetamine is half that of methylphenidate. Aside from the possibility of allergic reaction, the side effects to stimulants include loss of appetite, a failure to sleep well, and slower gain in weight and height.[346, 347] Intoxication with the medication may lead to irritability, tension, withdrawal from the environment, or even paranoia. In large overdoses, there may be gaze avoidance with stereotypic behavior and an autistic appearance.[348]

It is important to realize that medications given in the recommended dosages are not addicting.[349] Many physicians will prescribe stimulant medications only on school days or during times of excessive family stress such as large family gatherings, holidays, or cross country trips by automobile. This intermittent administration of medication may minimize the secondary effect of stimulant medication on weight and height reduction.[350] In addition, the administration of medication in the morning and at noontime may also minimize possible effects on sleep and on growth hormone secretion (growth hormone is secreted during the early stages of nocturnal sleep and is responsible for physical growth).[351] A recently marketed stimulant medication, pemoline (Cyclert®), and time release dextroamphetamine have the advantage of being given in a once a day dose schedule.[352]

Neurogenic Hyperactivity

Individuals who have experienced neurotoxic insults may have experienced insults in areas of the brain that control activity level as well as in areas that will produce motor or other developmental difficulties.[353] Since hyperactivity may be associated with an organic demonstrable historical event, e.g. meningoencephalitis, the term *organic driveness* has been applied to this group of children.[354] In its mildest form, the children would have soft neurological signs and some other signs of minimal developmental disabilities such as learning disability or difficulty with visual motor integrational skills or delays in neuromuscular coordination. It was this group of children that were labeled as minimal brain dysfunction in the past.[353, 356] Fortunately, this term is falling from use since it is a poorly descriptive term of multiple different problems (see Chapter 11). In this group of children, one may or may not be able to identify a neurotoxic event in their developmental, gestation, or perinatal history.

There are a group of children with a definite hard neurological sign and moderate to severe developmental disabilities who also have hyperactivity as part of their symptom complex. These individuals have suffered neurotoxic insults and have multiple developmental problems including hyperactivity. Again, the historical event may or may not be able to be identified in the child's history.

Children in the neurogenic group usually respond well to

stimulant medication.[357] However, many of these children represent complex problems, and there may be some psychosocial factors that also will affect their activity. This group of children with combined neurogenic and psychosocial factors are difficult to treat, requiring multiple treatment modalities.

Psychosocial Hyperactivity

Hyperactivity may be a manifestation of an emotional disturbance in a child who is neurologically intact and developmentally mature.[258] Hyperactivity may be a behavioral expression of anxiety. Hyperactivity is a common behavioral expression in children who are upset and worried. It may only be situationally manifested or in the case of the neurotic child, be present at all times. Hyperactive behavior may be seen in children who are in fact aggressive or psychotic, and during their periods of overactivity, they may destroy property and hurt other people or animals. Their behavior tends to be aggressive and destructive, but not consistently overenergetic during the twenty-four-hour period of their day.

Children who suffer emotional deprivation may also be hyperactive. They suffer from a lack of motivation to control their behavior and/or there may be obsessive pressure on the child to conform to a certain behavioral pattern. In these children, the emotional tensions that develop are relieved by a high activity level. Psychosocial hyperactivity can be divided into several categories (see Table XII), situational tension, childhood neurosis, childhood psychosis, and emotional deprivation.

Emotional Deprivation

As part of the normal maturation process, children learn to develop a readiness for conformity to environmental expectations.[258] If children do not develop inner emotional control to please their parents by receiving positive reinforcement and attention from them, they may not learn to inhibit their motor behavior. Whether they control their activity level or not they are still unacceptable to their parents or guardians. This can be understood by studying the activity level of the average two-year-old (the terrible twos).

The two-year-old is usually exceptionally active and would appear hyperactive as compared to a four-year-old child.[3] It is during this period that parents build in expectations for conformity in the control of their activity level. If the child learns to internalize the value that it is good to control his activity level, he will sit still and attend to tasks. However, if he does not incorporate this value, he will often present with hyperactive behavior. These children usually present in the three to six year age range. These children, like the child with primary or neurogenic hyperactivity, are in continual random motion and have a poor motivation for self control of their activity level.

Historical factors are important in helping to distinguish this group from the primary group. A history of physical neglect or abuse may be seen in these children. A history of failure to thrive in infancy or early childhood may have been seen. These children may show little or no separation anxiety. They may be friendly and smiling to everyone in their environment or they may be apathetically withdrawn from everyone in their environment. Later in life, there may be a history of wandering away from home and going into the neighbor's homes, having food with them without any interest in returning home. There may be a history of pica. There may be a history of a voracious appetite or thirst. These children may have had a history of prolonged self-stimulatory behavior such as rocking during the daytime (nighttime rocking has less significance). There may be the physical finding of a height and/or weight below the third percentile without a physical cause and in a family where the parents are of normal or above normal stature.

Typically, these children in later childhood and adolescence show a lack of motivation to behave in the schoolroom situation. They tend to be mistrustful and hostile towards authority figures. They test lower in IQ as a group, and they have poor control of their impulses. They may have temper tantrums and carry out acts for immediate gratification without concern for the consequences of their actions.

This type of hyperactivity may be seen with individuals who come from disorganized family units usually in the lower socioeconomic strata of society. Children reared in environments where there is a high amount of psychosocial disturbance such as alcoholism, neglect, brutality, delinquency, and crime grow up in an environment where people live from day to day. The children tend to have a low frustration level, are impulsive and have poor self control, and their dominant mode of action for tension reduction is in motor actions.

The treatment for children with deprivation as an etiology of their hyperactivity is to deal with the entire family and life situation. This may require interactional therapy involving the entire family unit. Sometimes with older children, individual therapy or individual counseling may be beneficial.

Situational Stress

The primary diagnostic clue for this category is the selective nature of the hyperactivity, its occurrence only in certain situations.[358] Children with situational stress induced hyperactivity have behavior that is characterized by being fidgety and squirming — having squirming motions while standing or sitting in one place. These children continually move their limbs around while attempting to be stationary or continually dart around the room much like the emotionally deprived child would behave.

It is important when one is obtaining the history of the child with hyperactivity to find out where the hyperactivity occurs. Many children are hyperactive in the classroom because of a variety of reasons, including peer pressure or inability to comprehend the classroom materials. Sometimes children may be bored because they are more advanced than their classmates and behave with hyperactivity. There are children who are only hyperactive in the home situation. This would relate to situational stress in their family unit.

In assessing children with situational stress hyperactivity, it is important to determine where they are hyperactive and to closely evaluate the stressful situation. Many children with hyperactivity in school will require psychometric testing to determine their mental abilities, while children who are hyperactive in the family unit should have the family unit structure carefully evaluated.

The obvious treatment for this type of hyperactivity is to determine the stressful stimulus in their environment and to take appropriate measures to eliminate the tension-inducing situation. This might include special educational classes, changing classrooms, or family counseling and therapy.

Childhood Neurosis

There are children who have the same behavioral manifestations as the child with situational tension hyperactivity, but their hyperactivity is not selectively restricted to certain high pressure situations.[358] These children are hyperactive in situations that, to the outside observer, should not be anxiety producing. These neurotic children require therapeutic intervention to alleviate their high level of anxiety.

The diagnosis of childhood neurosis with hyperactivity depends upon certain historical factors. Many of these children have an excessive sense of responsibility. These children may be labeled as worry-warts, children who are always concerned about what is happening to them or to their family members. These children may have had frequent somatic complaints such as tics, episodic abdominal pain, and episodic headaches. These children may have a history of exaggerated fears and excessive phobias, nightmares, or night terrors. These children may have shown school phobia early in their life. They may be excessively homesick when separated from their family unit for long periods of time.

Childhood Psychosis-Aggression

The hyperactivity of the psychotic or aggressive child is different than that seen with other forms of hyperactivity.[358] These children will have sudden erratic and changeable episodes of darting about from place to place and short attention span. These periods of overactive behavior may alternate with periods of inactivity and withdrawal. The reasons for the overactivity as well as for the withdrawal are not apparent to the observer and may only be appreciated by the child.

Aggressive children (and many psychotic children) will have a history of being destructive to property, animals, or individuals.

These episodes occur in response to internal stress. Children who are aggressive require psychiatric therapy.

Clues for determining childhood psychosis would include autistic behavior (Chapter 9). These children may show little or no emotional attachment to people. They may live in a world of their own that is not consistent with the reality of their environment. These children may lack social amenities. They may have episodes of unexpected or inappropriate smiling, laughter, or fears. There may be actual delusions or hallucinations. They may have episodes of inappropriate behavior. Psychotic children and aggressive children need referral to child psychiatrists and may require intensive therapy, anti-psychotic medications, or both.

Other Causes for Hyperactivity

The complaint of hyperactivity may be a manifestation of difficulty with a parent or teacher who cannot tolerate the normal activity level of a particular child. These children may present with a complaint of hyperactivity, but not appear hyperactive to other observers.

Hyperactivity may be a complication of certain medications. It has been reported as a side effect with the barbiturate medications.[219] It is also seen with antihistamines, antiasthmatics, and other drugs. A careful history of the onset of hyperactivity as well as the onset of treatment with various medications may be important in arriving at this conclusion.

Hyperactivity may be seen in children who require excessive outside stimulation such as those who have audiological or visual handicaps. These children may appear to behave with excessive motor activity in an attempt to increase their sensory input. Hyperactivity may also be seen with certain disease processes, such as hyperthyroidism. A careful physical examination and also laboratory tests may be necessary to determine these etiologies.

Since 1973, when Doctor Feingold[359] implicated food additives as an etiology in hyperactivity, there has been tremendous debate concerning the role of food additives in producing hyperactivity. There have been a variety of attempts to critically study the effect of food additives on activity levels.[360, 361] The results of these studies are inconsistent and contradictory. Knowing the high placebo response rate for treatment of hyperactivity makes one look with some skepticism upon reductions of activity levels in 30 to 40 percent of patients receiving dietary therapy.

There is some biochemical experimental support for specific food additives to alter central nervous system metabolism in such a way as to produce hyperactive behavior. There has been experimental evidence showing that the dopamine metabolic pathway is defective in *certain* hyperactive children.[362, 363] It has been shown in experimental rat studies that rats treated with a false dopamine neurotransmitter and then given red food coloring became hyperactive. Rats treated with just the false dopamine neurotransmitter also were hyperactive but their hyperactivity was intensified by the addition of food coloring.[364]

It may be that there is a small percentage of children who will respond to restrictions of food additives to their diet. From the experimental evidence, it would appear that the children who would respond are those who have some inherited or acquired change in their biochemical central nervous system state. The experimental evidence for food additives as an etiology in producing hyperactivity is somewhat tenuous, but there may be a small group of children who will respond with the elimination of food additives to control their high activity level.

Summary

Hyperactivity is a symptom that has many varied etiologies. The treatment depends upon the etiology of the hyperactivity. All children with hyperactive behavior should not be treated in the same manner. They require an extensive evaluation to determine whether their hyperactivity is constitutional or whether it is secondary to other factors. Most forms of hyperactivity are psychosocial in nature and would require some therapeutic intervention. There are many children who have a form of hyperactivity that will respond to treatment with stimulant medications. There are other children who might respond to various other forms of therapy. However, regardless of how the hyperactive child is treated medically, there is a very high placebo rate that may reflect an expectation from treatment, regardless of what the treatment is. Unfortunately, many children may suffer later in their life from inappropriate treatment and delay in intervention for other basic underlying problems.

Chapter 11

OTHER LEARNING AND
BEHAVIOR DISORDERS

THERE IS A LARGE BODY of literature concerning learning and behavior disorders.[365-374] Many investigators allege to define mechanisms of occurrence, etiology, and treatments. There are many attempts to correlate learning disorders with lesions seen in adults who suffer neurological insults or with animal experiments where certain areas are damaged. This has lead to many myths and nonscientific forms of therapy. Many concepts are based on the idea that other areas of the brain will *magically* take over for damaged function.

Much of the literature ignores the nature of injuries that affect developing nervous systems. In general, neurotoxic insults will produce diffuse injuries with certain areas involved with greater severity. The result is usually a developmental lag in one or several areas. In these cases, function develops, but it develops at a slower rate than normal and usually does not achieve the normal level of performance (Chapter 1). Genetic factors should also be considered, since we each inherit our own native intelligence.[375, 376] This native intelligence involves differences in substrata of intelligence; we may inherit a greater facility in some areas than in others.

It is interesting to reflect on changes in society's attitude. Three decades ago, if a child was not succeeding in school, he was termed *slow*. Today he is termed *learning disabled*. A term or label like *learning disability* implies a defined condition with remedial treatment, when, in many instances, no form of treatment will be capable of producing an increase in that individual's intellect.

Likewise we are all born with certain personality characteristics.[377] Environment will influence the development of our personality, but each one of us has an inherent personality makeup. It is interesting to visit a newborn nursery and observe

151

the difference in infants and how they respond to people, their frustration tolerance, their irritability, and their response to the environment. Even as a newborn, individuals tend to have different personality structures.

Just as neurotoxic insults are capable of affecting our motor, speech, or intellectual development, neurotoxic insults are capable of altering areas of our brain that control our personality, activity level, frustration tolerance, etc.[378-381] Developmental lags in personality may be seen. This can be reflected in the intellectually delayed child whose personality stages are also delayed. Many of these children behave like chronologically younger children. They often play with chronologically younger aged children.

The attempt to apply the medical model of illness to learning and behavior disorders has also contributed to our misunderstanding of these problems. This approach to a problem involves finding historical factors, positive physical findings, and a pathological area of disease and then applying a diagnostic term.

There are no definite consistent historical factors to support a diagnosis of a learning or behavior problem. However, the cadence of the individual's developmental milestones may be important in deciding if one is dealing with a learning disability. One would look for prenatal, perinatal, or postnatal catastrophes that may have been responsible for neurotoxic insults, as well as looking for acquired illnesses such as encephalitis or meningitis, which may also have produced neurologic damage. There are some familial factors that are important. Occasionally learning, particularly reading disabilities, may be seen in male family members of certain pedigrees. The intellectual quotient of the parents and the educational level of the parent may also be informative.

The search for physical signs in individuals with learning and behavior problems has lead to the search for soft neurological signs or signs of immaturity of the nervous system. Soft neurological signs are findings that may be normal in a younger child, but, in the course of maturation, should have disappeared or signs that can be brought out only by special neurological maneuvers. The finding of hard neurological signs may support the diagnosis of a learning or behavioral problem. However, one does not always find soft or hard neurological signs in these children.

Studies that hope to define the area in the brain that has been pathologically affected in most cases have been disappointing. In severe injury, such as those seen with congenital malformations of the brain, multiple areas of pathology may be defined. Although, in individuals with subtler learning and behavioral difficulties, one often sees no evidence of focal pathology on postmortem examination of the brain, recent studies indicate subtle anatomical differences from normal.[382, 383] Pathological injuries to developing nervous systems are different than injuries to a mature nervous system; when an area is destroyed in an adult, it is immediately reflected in a loss of prior function. Pathological processes that affect the mature nervous system are also different in that adults are more prone to processes that will focally destroy parts of their nervous system.

Finally, the desire to label individuals as having a particular entity has further contributed to confusion and mismanagement in the field of learning and behavioral disorders. Application of terminology such as minimal brain dysfunction and dyslexia implies a certain finality to the evaluation process. Unfortunately, terms such as these are only generally symptomatically descriptive and not specifically descriptive of the individual child's difficulty.[1] For example, the term *dyslexia* merely implies difficulty reading. It gives no clue as to the etiology of the reading difficulty. The therapy for reading disability depends on the etiology. The application of terms such as these tends to lump individuals into treatment programs that are not applicable for all individuals with that disability.

Minimal Brain Dysfunction

The term *minimal brain dysfunction* is an outgrowth of the term *minimal cerebral dysfunction*.[384] Minimal cerebral dysfunction was first used in the late 1950s. Investigators began to notice that there were children who were hyperactive, were clumsy (had a delay in their neuromuscular coordinative skills), and had difficulty learning in school. In addition, many of these children had soft neurological signs.[385] Although the term implied some finality diagnostically, it actually contributed little to care of children with these difficulties.

The term *minimal brain dysfunction* may have contributed in a negative fashion to the care and treatment of children with these problems.[386] Since some forms of hyperactivity are known to respond to stimulant medications (Chapter 10), children with other difficulties, such as delayed coordinative skills or learning disabilities, were then assumed to be responsive to such medications. This form of thinking led to the inference that many of the factors described as minimal brain dysfunction would also respond to stimulant medications. This led to 5 to 10 percent of individuals in elementary school systems being treated with stimulant medications for behavior disorders.[387] Clearly, certain children with hyperactivity (Chapter 10) will respond to stimulant medication, but children with only delays in neuromuscular coordinative skills and only learning disabilities do not improve with stimulant medication.

Another difficulty with the term *minimal brain dysfunction* is the qualifier minimal. Although there have been volumes written on minimal brain dysfunction, how minimal is minimal?[385, 388, 389] Where one draws the line in terms of degree of handicap has never been elucidated. In counseling parents it is often kinder to euphemistically term the child *minimal brain dysfunction* than to term him *retarded* or *cerebral palsied*. This is because the other terms carry with them negative stigmata whereas the term *minimal brain dysfunction* implies that there is only some mild difficulty with the child. Because of the nonspecificity of the term, it is now falling from disuse in the medical community. It is to the child's advantage for him to be descriptively termed as a child with hyperactivity or learning disabilities or delayed neuromuscular coordinative skills or any combination of the above rather than labeling him minimal brain dysfunction.

Attention Deficit Disorder

With the disuse of the term *minimal brain dysfunction,* another term has crept into the literature, that of *attention deficit disorder.*[338, 339] Unlike minimal brain dysfunction, attention deficit disorder describes children who have a high activity level and/or an inability to focus their attention on tasks at hand. This term would overlap with the description of primary hyperactivity and hyperactivity secondary to neurogenic factors associated with soft neurological signs (Chapter 10). The important implication of the term attention deficit disorder is that there may be children who do not overtly appear hyperactive, but, when required to sit and complete a given task, they are unable to focus their attention on the task at hand, being easily distracted by any extraneous stimuli. Because of their inability to attend to tasks or symbols at hand there may be some difficulty with serial ordering and/or attending to reading whole words.

Delayed Neuromuscular Coordination

Children with a delay in neuromuscular coordinative skills appear clumsy. This condition has been labeled as the *clumsy child syndrome*.[390] These children lag in acquiring the skill with their fine neuromuscular coordination that other children achieve at the same chronological ages during the developmental process. Symptoms these children may manifest include: difficulty coloring in the lines, difficulty in manipulating scissors, a delay in tying shoe laces, inability to succeed in games requiring coordinative skills such as hopping, skipping, catching, and kicking. These children can be identified by using the testing of neuromuscular coordinative skills outlined in Table II.

These children represent developmental lags in the acquisition of fine motor skills. Therapy should be directed at building their confidence rather than building the expectation that therapeutic programs will hasten their neuromuscular development. This can best be accomplished by giving them fine coordinative tasks they are capable of doing and advancing them to more sophisticated tasks as their nervous system matures.

Children in this group may have some difficulty in acquiring right-left orientation by seven years of age[9, 10] and along with this may have some difficulty with serial ordering items, e.g. they may mistake 579 for 597. This may also be reflected in spelling errors. There is another group of children with delayed neuromuscular coordinative skills who are important to identify. They are children who are unable to carry out rapid-fire commands by seven years of age (see Table II).[9, 10] The anticipation of parents and teachers is that by the time the child is in the first grade or beginning of the second grade he should be able to carry out a series of commands in succession. However, these children with an immaturity in their coordinative skills may be unable to accomplish this act. It is important to identify these children because they may be labeled as obstinate or as behavioral problems or as children who do not complete their work in the classroom. They are not volitionally being obstinate, forgetful, or lazy, but they lack the ability to carry out more than one command at a time.

After this problem is identified in the child, the parents and teachers can be instructed to address the child with one step rather than multiple step commands. Thus, much of the anxiety in the child and much of the interaction difficulties between child and parent or child and teacher can be eliminated. For example, a child with this disability who is told in the classroom to open his desk, take out his blue book, turn to page 57, and start problem 9 is fortunate if he can open his desk and find his blue book let alone turn to the appropriate page and start the appropriate problem. The child is bewildered as to what is happening and does not understand why he is being chastised for asking his neighbor what to do next.

These children in the home situation will have difficulty remembering to do the same tasks every day, e.g. taking the trash out each morning on the way to school. These children must be reminded on a daily basis to do their tasks. When the parent gives the child too many commands in succession they will not be accomplished. For example, if a parent tells his child to go up to his room, make his bed, and straighten up his room, the child is fortunate to make it to his room let alone make his bed and straighten up the area. This child should be told to go to his room, once he is there told to make his bed, and, after his bed is made, told to straighten his room. Handled in this manner the negative self image that these children may acquire can be attenuated and the feeling that they are behavioral disorders can be eliminated.

Handedness

Much has been written concerning the higher frequency of left handedness in children with learning and behavioral disorders as well as in individuals in institutions for the developmentally disabled or the psychiatrically disabled.[369-371, 391] There are a number of individuals who are normal and are left handed. However, there is an increase in the incidence of left-handed developmentally disabled individuals. This can be explained in the following manner: if the nervous system experiences a neurotoxic insult that strikes the system generally, but tends to involve one hemisphere with greater severity than the other, since these insults would be random, the frequency of affecting the left hemisphere would be as high as injuries affecting the right hemisphere. As a result, an increased number of neurologically damaged individuals will show left handedness. Individuals who are left handed and also show signs of right body dysfunctions are at risk for having developmental disabilities or learning and behavior problems but their risk is the same as someone who is right handed and shows signs of left sided dysfunction.

Specific Learning Disabilities

Children may have difficulty learning in school as the result of environmental, emotional, physical, or neurodevelopmental difficulties. Usually, in the evaluation of a child with a learning disability, it is necessary to involve an interdisciplinary team to successfully arrive at the etiology of learning disability. The American Academy of Pediatrics Council on Child Health has defined a learning disability.[392] In their definition, the child with a true learning disability has an average or above average intelligence. They have specific learning or behavioral abnormalities. These abnormalities are characterized by mild to severe deficits with auditory perception, visual perception association, conceptualization, language competence, motor function or with con-

trol of attention and impulse. Children with a general depression in intellectual function (mentally retarded) are excluded
from their definition. Also, children with sensory, visual, auditory or motor handicaps or emotional disturbances are excluded
from their definition.

Since it is implicit in this definition of learning disability that
intelligence be average or above, it is important to obtain an
accurate assessment of intellectual quotient based on standard-
ized testing.[393-399] Not only would one look at the overall score of
the individual's intelligence test, but one should look at the
scatter of scores on the various subtests. Intelligence really can be
broken down into many areas including verbal ability, performance ability, numerical ability, abstract reasoning abilities, ability
to discern forms in space, and the ability to determine serial
ordering or symbols. It is important to ascertain if there are
discrepancies in certain of these areas and not in others. Also, it is
important to determine if there is a discrepancy between the
child's verbal abilities and performance abilities.[400-403]

Over the last decades there has been increasing sophistication
in the development of tests that evaluate a child's ability to
process stimuli and information introduced to him via auditory
or tactile routes.[405-410] It is possible to identify children who have
difficulties in processing in the various modalities. What is usually found with these tests is that the individual performs at an age
less than his chronological age in specific processing skills, again
pointing to a developmental lag in these areas.

It is important to identify children who have specific inabilities
to process or to learn via auditory or symbolic forms of teaching.
Once these children are identified, their educational program
can be altered so that they are given the bulk of their instruction
in their nonhandicapped areas. However, it is unfortunate that
in many instances it is difficult if not impossible to teach in
alternate ways. It is the globally intellectually bright child who is
able to circumvent his specific processing difficulty and circumvent his handicap. The child with the borderline or low-normal
intelligence, who also has a learning disability, has limited other
resources to draw upon and often has difficulty learning via
alternate methods.[412]

Reading Disability

Reading is a complicated act of cognitive processing. Reading can be broken down into several different functions.[413-415] A person must be able to discriminate forms, to discriminate their sequence, to discriminate their orientation in space, to be able to break a word into speech sounds and put it together, to be able to remember the symbolic meaning of letters, to have the appropriate attention to concentrate on the whole word rather than just the first portion of it, and must have achieved a certain developmental level in order to process symbols. There are so many factors involved in the process of reading and defects in any one of these areas may produce inability to read appropriately for age. Calling someone who is unable to read a dyslexic really achieves nothing.[1] The term *dyslexia* only means difficulty reading. It does not imply a one term, one etiology condition.

All children who have difficulty reading should *not* be treated for their disability in the same manner.[416-418] A child may not be able to concentrate on his words so that he will make his judgement on the first portion of a word (this child will often read *these* and *there* and *those* as the same or interchangeable words). In order to correct this deficit, the child's attention may have to be improved with medication or he may have to be taught reading in a way where only the whole word appears in front of him rather than an entire line of words. This way he learns to set a cadence to his eye movement that will encompass the entire word rather than looking at just the beginning of the word. This problem requires a very different treatment than the child who is developmentally delayed in acquiring reading skills. These children will commonly reverse their letters.

When it was in vogue to teach very young children in the three to five age bracket to read in the hopes of improving their overall reading abilities and intellectual performance, it was found that three to five year olds commonly will reverse letters and symbols.[419] These children were reading *was* as *saw* or *saw* as *was*, and reversed the *e*'s as *ɘ*'s and the *s*'s as *ƨ*'s. To them the mirror image of letters was not significant because they would perceive the letter when it was oriented in the traditional fashion or not. There only was difficulty with letters such as *b*'s and *d*'s and *p*'s and *q*'s where the mirror symbol has a different meaning. By the time these children were seven years of age, they were no longer reversing their letters. It only is abnormal for children to reverse letters after the age of seven years.

It was found that by the time the children who were started reading at three to five years of age reached the second to third grade that they were reading at the same level as their peers who started learning to read in the first grade, thus emphasizing that it is impossible to have a nervous system mature faster than it is destined. Ultimately, the children who started in early reading programs did not differ in their reading achievement from the children who started in reading programs at the traditional age. Children with delays in acquiring reading skills on a developmental basis will reverse letters past the age of seven and will often read mirror words such as *was-saw* or mirror letters such as *p-q* and *b-d*. Since this is a developmental problem these children need to be identified and treated by addressing their reading tasks to their developmental level.

Aberrant Behavioral Patterns

Behavioral disorders in the developmentally disabled involve an interplay between neurogenic factors, psychosocial factors, and inherent personality factors. Children suffering psychological insults may regress or become fixed in a behavioral stage.

Neurotoxic insults are capable of producing damage to behavioral areas of the brain and in doing so may cause a slow maturation of an individual's behavior.[378-381] This will result in a persistence of behavioral patterns at developmental levels below the person's chronological age. An individual may not progress beyond certain stages in his personality development and be left with permanent functioning at a lower level of behavior. Impaired individuals will spend longer periods of time in each behavioral stage. Because of certain environmental factors, they may persist in a behavioral pattern even though they are capable of achieving a higher level of behavioral performance.

This concept can be exemplified with the temper tantrums that one often sees in normal two year olds.[3] Parents ignore these outbursts, give the child negative reinforcement for the behavior and the child learns not to have temper tantrums. This is also true for biting behavior, body rocking, and head banging.[420] Most one and one-half to two-year-olds at some point in their life will bite either themselves or other individuals. They learn very quickly that this is not acceptable behavior and learn to control this impulse. Unfortunately, many children with developmental disabilities who exhibit behavioral abnormalities of biting or temper tantrum outbursts will receive reinforcement for their negative behavior by getting attention from those around them. One of the hallmarks of behavior modification therapy is that negative behavior is *not* reinforced. Many individuals inadvertently reinforce negative behavior by giving the child attention only when he has abnormal behavior. Behavior modification techniques may be quite successful in modifying episodic temper tantrum outbursts and episodic biting behavior.[421, 425]

Many children with developmental disabilities are emotionally deprived and/or deprived of sensory input. Individuals who lack sensory input from visual or auditory stimuli may be hyperactive or may exhibit forms of self-stimulatory behavior almost in an attempt to compensate for lack of stimulation received by their sense organs. Behavior such as rocking and head banging is not uncommonly seen in individuals with sensory organ deprivation. This is also true for individuals who suffer from emotional deprivation. They may rely on self-stimulation from rocking, head banging, masturbation, or biting themselves to compensate for lack of warmth and attention from caretakers. Lesch-Nyhan is a condition, diagnosed by high serum uric acid levels, where self mutilation is characteristic.[426] Behavior modification techniques for nonorganic forms of self stimulatory behavior can be successful.

Behavioral outbursts are not uncommon in young children. They often are provoked by siblings or by peers. Children who have behavioral outbursts may bite and scream and damage items in their vicinity. This behavior in someone who is thirty-five pounds and three feet tall will not produce much damage to the adults or to material in his area, but an individual who developmentally is functioning at a behavior level of three years, who is 6 feet and 250 pounds may inflict considerable damage to people, equipment, and property in his area.

If the patient with a developmental disability has a behavioral outburst it is important to determine what was the provoking cause. If there were no external provoking causes for behavioral outbursts, the child should be evaluated for the possibility of psychosis where the provoking stimulus for the behavioral outburst may have come from within and was not related to his environment.

Individuals who have temporal lobe seizures may have outbursts of what appear to be behavioral abnormalities as a manifestation of seizure.[23] Individuals who have temporal lobe seizures manifested by behavioral outbursts often have some autonomic nervous system dysfunction associated with their episodes, such as reddening of the face or blank staring. They will repeat the same stereotypic acts (whether it be running and punching a hole in the wall or tearing their clothes) during each episode. Provided no one interferes with their automatic activity, the person will not harm other individuals. If, however, a caretaker tries to interfere with their activity they are likely to be the brunt of injury. Individuals who have temporal lobe seizures are often somnolent after the event, usually have no memory for what has transpired, and have no remorse for the event (Chapter 7).

A form of psychosis that may be associated with behavorial outbursts is manic depressive psychosis.[427] This is a familial condition, and individuals who are afflicted with it will have periods of withdrawal or depression that may alternate with periods of grandiose hyperactive manic style behavior (Chapter 12).

Summary

Children with developmental disabilities have an increased incidence of learning disabilities and behavioral disorders. Since individuals who have suffered some neurotoxic insult may have learning disabilities and/or behavioral disorders, these conditions can be viewed in a neurodevelopmental perspective. It is important to identify their developmental nature. Once viewed as a developmental rather than a static disability, appropriate treatment programs can be selected for the achievement of realistic goals and objectives.

Chapter 12

DRUGS AFFECTING BEHAVIOR

O VER THE PAST THREE DECADES there have been significant advances in the use of medication to alter behavior.[423, 429] These advances have resulted in more effective treatment for patients. As a result of these advances, more individuals with psychoses or behavioral problems have been able to function outside of institutions. There has been a decrease in the need for physical restraints. The effective use of antidepressant medication has diminished the need for electroconvulsive therapy.

Medications that alter behavior have biochemical effects within the central nervous system.[430-433] The elucidation of these effects has led to more research into the organic basis of abnormal behavior. As a result, there has been increasing evidence that psychoses, schizophrenia and manic-depressive, have a genetic basis, resulting from inherited enzyme defects in specific biochemical pathways of the brain metabolism.[434-440] The effectiveness of the psychopharmacologic agents in altering behavior has been the impetus for the introduction of new medications to relieve behavioral and psychotic disorders.

Certain medications have been abused through illicit street usage leading to addiction and dependency. Hence, there is some concern by the lay population about their use in patients.[441] The addicting dosage of most medication is three to six times the normal prescribed therapeutic dosage. When the medications are judiciously prescribed, they are compensating for biochemical defects in brain metabolism rather than causing the untoward metabolic derangements that are seen with street abuse.

There is confusion in terminology concerning the usage of the term *tranquilizer*.[442] Because anti-anxiety medications produce sedation and a diminution of anxiety and tension, they are commonly referred to as tranquilizers. Pharmacologically, the only true tranquilizers are the anti-psychotic medications. In an

164

attempt to differentiate the two groups, the term *minor tranquilizer* has been applied to the anti-anxiety agents and the term *major tranquilizer* applied to the anti-psychotic agents. However, pharmacologically, the anti-anxiety agents belong to the sedative-hypnotic group of medications, and the anti-psychotic medications are the only true tranquilizers.

The medications that alter behavior can be divided into the following groups: anti-anxiety agents, anti-psychotic agents, anti-manic agents, anti-depressants, and central nervous system stimulants. These categories will be discussed in generalities. Medications will vary in their abilities to produce the effects and side effects seen in each group.

Anti-Anxiety Medications

Pharmacologically, anti-anxiety medications[432, 442-443] are classified among the sedative-hypnotic medications. In general, the medications in this category (see Table XIII) will reduce anxiety and tension when administered in small dosage. In large doses, they will produce sleep (hypnotic effective). In larger doses, they will produce a general anesthesia, and, in exceptionally large doses, they will produce a depression of vital brain center functions causing respiratory depression and death. With repeated usages, higher dosages are required to produce the same effects for relief of anxiety or induction of sleep. Inappropriately used, they may become habituating and cause physical dependence.

These medications cause a relief of psychological tension and anxiety and may produce euphoria. Casual usage without adequate physician supervision has resulted in habituation to these medications. Once a person has been habituated to these medications, the abrupt withdrawal may produce a withdrawal state. Abrupt withdrawal may lead to hyperexcitability, autonomic nervous system stimulation, convulsions, delirium tremors, psychosis, and even death. Whenever someone has been maintained on sedative-hypnotic medication, they must be gradually tapered to prevent the appearance of the withdrawal state. Fortunately, the anticonvulsant action of the anti-anxiety drugs does not require increasing dosages for maintenance of control

Table XIII
COMMONLY PRESCRIBED ANTI-ANXIETY MEDICATIONS

Alcohols
    Chloral hydrate
    Ethanol
    Ethchlorvynold (Placidyl®)
Antihistamines
    Diphenhydramine (Benadryl®)
    Hydroxyzine hydrochloride (Atarax®, Vistaril®)
    Promethazine hydrochloride (Phenergan®)
Barbiturates
    Amobarbital (Amytal®)
    Mephobarbital (Mebaral®)
    Pentobarbital (Nembutal®)
    Phenobarbital (Luminal®)
    Primidone (Mysoline®)
    Secobarbital (Seconal®)
    Thiopental (Pentothal®)
Benzodiazepines
    Clonazepam (Clonapen®)
    Chlordiazepoxide (Librium®)
    Diazepam (Valium®)
    Flurazepam (Dalmane®)
    Oxazepam (Serax®)
Cyclic ether
    Paraldehyde
Dicarbamates
    Carisoprodol (Rela®, Soma®)
    Meprobamate (Equanil®, Miltown®)
Piperidinediones
    Glutethimide (Doriden®)
    Methyprylon (Noludar®)
Quinazolone
    Methaqualone (Quaalude®)

(see Chapter 7). The anticonvulsant property of these medications will be maintained with consistent dosage administration.

The anti-anxiety medications are thought to act in the central nervous system by producing a generalized depression in neuronal cell function with specific effect in the reticular activating system of the brain. The reticular activating system is responsible for our awakefulness. There is extensive individual variation to the effects of the anti-anxiety medications. The most commonly used medication with which most of us are familiar is alcohol. There is a great variation among individuals in their ability to tolerate the effects of alcohol and the amount required to produce side effects.

Anti-anxiety medications cause sedation with a decreased responsiveness to external stimuli. Drowsiness occurs and, if sufficient dosage is administered, sleep will occur. Prior to the induction of sleep, individuals will become ataxic (unsteady), and nystagmus (jerkiness of eye movement) may also be seen. There is a dysinhibition of higher cortical centers with larger dosages and a release of phylogenetically more primitive forms of activity so that the individual may lose the constant fine control of his behavior. In larger dosages, the person may appear to be euphoric. All these effects are accompanied by an impairment in judgement and a loss of self control. In some individuals there may be a transient period of excitement.

The excitement was initially thought to be a paradoxical effect of the medication, but actually is consistent with its effect on central nervous system depression. Since action of neuronal cells is maintained in balance by factors that cause stimulation and factors that cause inhibition, individuals in whom there is excitation will have an increase in the depression of the cellular inhibitors allowing the cellular exciters to temporarily exert greater action. With higher dosages of medication, the exciters will become inhibited and the patient will show central nervous system depression and, in massive doses, anesthesia. Along with these effects, there is some analgesic effect so that the person's perception of pain is diminished. The narcotics are much more effective in inducing analgesia than the anti-anxiety agents.

Along with their effect on the brain is an effect on the polysynaptic reflexes of the spinal cord, causing a depression in polysynaptic circuits inducing muscle relaxation.

Anti-Psychotic Medications

The anti-psychotic medications[432, 442, 444, 445] (see Table XIV) are pharmacologically the only true tranquilizers. In contrast to the anti-anxiety agents they do not induce anesthesia. Patients can be aroused after administration of exceptionally high dosages of the anti-psychotic medications. These medications are not habituating. They are convulsant and may precipitate seizures. They cause side effects involving the extra-pyramidal system (the system that controls the fine tuning of motor movement). Their primary use is in treatment of psychosis.

Table XIV
COMMONLY PRESCRIBED ANTI-PSYCHOTIC MEDICATION

Butyrophenone
  Haloperidol (Haldol®)
Phenothiazine
  Chlorpromazine (Thorazine®)
  Fluphenazine (Prolixin®, Permitil®)
  Prochlorperazine (Compazine®)
  Promazine (Sparine®)
  Thioridazine (Mellaril®)
  Trifluoperazine (Stelazine®)
Thioxanthenes
  Chlorprothixene (Taractan®)
  Thiothixine (Navane®)

The type of sedation that anti-psychotic medications induce is very distinctive, will not progress to anesthesia, but produces a state of ineffectiveness or apathy. There is a retardation in motor activity from which arousal by ordinary stimuli can occur despite even high dosages of this medication. When a psychotic patient becomes anxious and combative because of psychotic episodes, the anti-psychotic tranquilizers can be used to treat this form of anxiety. Sedatives may also be used to control an acute psychotic event.

Habituation and dependence to these medications do not occur. Many individuals who take them do not like the feeling of apathy and ineffectiveness and may attempt to voluntarily discontinue their medication despite the control of their psychotic symptomatology. Although the behavioral effect of the medication is to reduce the activity level of the patient, neurophysiologically, the medication is acting in a stimulating capacity. This is reflected with their capacity in large dosages to precipitate convulsions.

The limbic system (controlling centers for emotion and behavior) is sensitive to the anti-psychotic medications. Also, the diencephalon and the hypothalamus (control centers of our endocrine and autonomic nervous system) are sensitive. This accounts for some side effects such as dry mouth, large pupils, failure to accommodate for near vision, constipation, and tachycardia. Postural hypotension may occur, leading to episodes of fainting and precipitous falls in blood pressure. There may be a decrease in body temperature and decrease in shivering. Endocrine-metabolic side effects include a gain in weight, menstrual irregularity, impotence, and lactation.

There are several possible effects on the extra-pyramidal system (movement control system). Individuals may have Parkinsonian-like symptoms including mask-like facies, muscular rigidity, fine resting tremor, and shuffling gait. There may be akathisias, which is a feeling of restlessness and a compulsion to move. Patients manifesting this side effect may walk impatiently, tap their foot, or appear to have restless limbs. There may be dystonia (involuntary movements about large muscle groups causing the patient to assume bizarre postures). There may be oculogyric crises. These potential movement side effects may be reversed with discontinuation or decrease in the medication. The potential problem of tardiff dyskinesia may remain despite discontinuation of the anti-psychotic tranquilizer. Tardiff dyskinesias are involuntary discoordinated rhythmical movements that often occur about the tongue, lips, face or jaw.

Other side effects include pigmentation of the skin on body parts exposed to the sun, pigmentary deposits in the anterior chamber of the lens leading to cataract formation, and a pigmentary retinopathy where pigment becomes deposited in the retina leading to impairment of vision. There may be jaundice secondary to hepatic biliary obstruction and a photosensitive eczemoid-like rash.

In spite of all the potential side effects, these medications do continue in common usage because they actively ameliorate the symptoms of psychosis. They will reduce the excitement and control the hostile aggressive behavior. They will suppress the symptoms of psychotic ideation. These medications will reduce the hallucinatory phenomena that psychotic patients experience. In addition, they can be used for problems of emotional instability and abnormal behavior associated with chronic brain syndromes.

Anti-Manic Medications[427, 432, 442, 444, 445, 447, 448]

Manic-depressive psychosis is a condition in which individuals experience periods of disassociation with reality. During these periods they may behave in either a manic fashion, where they are excitable and grandiose, or in a depressed fashion, where they are withdrawn.[427] There are individuals with manic-depressive psychosis who are unipolar and will experience episodes in only one of these phases, either the manic or the depressive. Individuals who will experience periods of mania alternating with periods of depression are called bipolar. Before the advent of lithium carbonate there was no medication that was consistently effective in treating the manic-depressive psychosis. Lithium is not effective in the management of a person in an agitated acute manic episode. These individuals will respond to treatment with anti-psychotic tranquilizers. Lithium will be effective in the manic phase of this illness after five to ten days of treatment. The primary usefulness of lithium is in the prophylactic control of manic-depressive psychosis. Although the mode of action of lithium has not been completely elucidated, it does affect the sodium-potassium balance system responsible for neuronal cell excitability.

The mild side effects of lithium include nausea and fine tremor. More severe side effects include anorexia, vomiting, diarrhea, increase in liquid consumption, coarsening of tremor, muscular weakness and twitching, general body sedation, and hypotonia. More severe side effects would include stupor, confusional-like state, seizures, coma, and death. The severity of the side effects directly relate with the serum level of lithium. In managing patients, lithium serum levels are maintained in the 0.6 to 1.2 milliequivalents/liter range. Toxic symptomatology appears to arise if the serum blood level exceeds 1.6 milliequivalents/liter. Because of the potential for side effects on renal or cardiovascular function patients with cardiovascular disease or renal impairment should not be given lithium carbonate. Patients maintained on lithium should have periodic evaluations of their renal function and their cardiac status.

Anti-Depressant Medications[432, 442, 444, 445]

Most depressions are exogenous. They are the result of external psychosocial factors. Factors such as loss are the primary cause of exogenous depression. Endogenous depressions occur

Table XV
COMMONLY PRESCRIBED ANTI-DEPRESSANT MEDICATIONS

Amitriptyline (Elavil®)
Desmethylimipramine (Norpramin®, Pertofrane®)
Imipramine (Tofranil®)
Nortriptyline (Aventyl®)
Protriptyline (Vivactil®)

in individuals where no external factors of stress or loss have precipitated the depressive episode. Individuals who have endogenous depression tend to have diminution in their motor activity. There appears to be little or no hostility, self commendation, or agitation. Some biochemical abnormalities have been seen in the nervous systems of individuals with endogenous depression, and there may be a genetic predisposition to endogenous depression.[442, 445]

Endogenous depressions respond well to anti-depressant medications (see Table XV). Pharmacologically, these medications are similar in structure to the anti-psychotic tranquilizers. They will produce a sedation similar to that produced by the anti-psychotic medications. In addition, patients may note weakness, drowsiness, or increase in subjective tension, tremulousness, visual hallucinations, or agitation. The autonomic nervous system side effects seen with anti-psychotic tranquilizers may occur with the anti-depressants. Side effects such as dry mouth, postural hypotension, blurred vision, and constipation are seen. Metabolic effects such as weight gain, edema, and cardiac arrhythmias may occur. In large doses, anti-depressants may induce severe cardiac arrhythmia resulting in death.

Despite the potential side effects these medications are used in the treatment of endogenous depression because they appear to correct the biochemical abnormality in these conditions, bringing the person back to a state of well being. Their use in exogenous depression is limited.

Stimulant Medications

Stimulant medications[348, 432, 442] (Table XVI) induce wakefulness, decrease fatigue, and induce euphoria. In larger doses,

Table XVI

COMMONLY PRESCRIBED STIMULANT MEDICATION

Amphetamine (Benzedine®)
Dextroamphetamine (Dexedrine®)
Methamphetamine (Desoxyn®, Methedrine®)
Methylphenidate (Ritalin®)
Pemoline (Cyclert®)

they may induce anxiety and in even larger doses, produce hyperexcitability, insomnia, or psychosis. Pharmacologically, these are related to the ephedrine class of sympathomimetic agents. Therefore they have side effects on our autonomic nervous system including tremulousness, dry mouth, awareness of the heart beat, increase in dreaming during sleep, and decrease in sleep. There may be increase in blood pressure and pulse and pupillary dilatation. Although they may decrease the appetite, the effect on appetite is not stable so that in time a person will develop a tolerance to the medication's appetite suppressive effect. In approximately six to eight weeks, it will be ineffective as an appetite control agent. The primary usefulness of CNS stimulants for developmentally disabled is in the treatment of hyperkinetic children (Chapter 10). These medications also have some usefulness in the treatment of narcoleptics.

PHENYLKETONURIA AND OTHER AMINOACIDOPATHIES[449-451]

Aminoacidopathy	*Abnormal Enzyme*	*Metabolic Disturbance*
Defects of Phenylalanine & Tyrosine Metabolism		
Phenylalanine		
Neonatal hyperphenylalaninemia	(?) phenylalanine hydroxylating system immaturity	Phenylalanine in blood, urine usually negative
Classical phenylketonuria	Phenylalanine hydroxylase (only trace activity)	Phenylalanine in blood and urine, phenylpyruric, phenyllactic, phenylacetic and hydroxyphenylacotic acids in urine.
Atypical phenylketonuria	Partial defect in phenylalanine hydroxylase.	Same as classical but usually smaller amounts.
Transient phenylketonuria	Partial defect in phenylalanine hydroxylase, may be other factors involved.	Same as classical.
Benign hyperphenylalaninemia	Phenylalanine hydroxylase	Phenylalanine in blood and urine.

Treatment	Clinical Features	Comment
None.	Primarily in premature infants. May be a normal transient phenomenon in newborns.	Often occur with hypertyrosinemia. Benign condition.
Dietary restriction of phenylalanine to 250 to 500 mg per day.	Seizures, mental retardation, eczema, light hair and skin.	Must keep plasma phenylalanine below 16 mg/100 ml to prevent retardation, treatment may be stopped after age four years without deterioration, musty odor to urine.
Dietary restriction of phenylalanine, 500 mg per day to tolerance.	Mental retardation (usually less severe than classical).	Same as classical.
Same as classical.	Same as classical.	Must monitor carefully for change in status to normal after several months or years of age and adjust diet accordingly.
None.	Normal.	May be result of complex gene and/or cofactor interactions.

Aminoacidopathy	Abnormal Enzyme	Metabolic Disturbance
Offspring of maternal phenylketonuria	No deficiency (if heterozygote)	None after birth.

Tyrosine

Aminoacidopathy	Abnormal Enzyme	Metabolic Disturbance
Neonatal tyrosinemia	p-hydroxyphenylpyruvate hydroxylase	Tyrosine, pHPPA, pHPLA, pHPAA and N-acetyltyrosine in urine, tyrosine in blood.
Tyrosinosis (Medes)	(?) L-tyrosine pyruvate aminotransferase	pHPPA
Hypertyrosinemia (Oregon type)	Cytosoltyrosine aminotransferase (hepatic)	Tyrosine in urine and blood, pHPPA, pHPLA and pHPAA in urine.
Hereditary tyrosinemia	p-hydroxyphenylpyruvate hydroxylase	Tyrosine and methionine in blood. Generalized aminoaciduria with increased tyrosine in urine.
Alcaptonuria	Homogentistic acid oxidase	Homogentistic acid in urine and blood.

Treatment	Clinical Features	Comment
None.	Congenital malformations, developmental and mental retardation.	Treatment of mother during gestation with low phenylalanine diet.
Ascorbic acid and low protein diet may be helpful.	Usually benign, lethargy in premature, ? IQ deficits.	Usually benign. Occurs primarily in premature infants.
None	Myasthenia gravis (? incidental findings)	Postulated defect locally in kidney.
None effective	Multiple congenital anomalies, severe mental retardation.	
Dietary restriction of tyrosine and methionine and phenylalanine.	Hepatic cirrhosis, renal tubular failure, porphuric-like state, Fanconi syndrome, vomiting, diarrhea, failure to thrive, hypoglycemia, glycosuria.	Acute form may have liver failure and death in first year of life and cabbage-like odor to urine. Chronic form may have hepatic, cirrhosis and classical clinical features.
None late in disease (?), phenylalanine and tyrosine dietary restriction to 200 to 500 mg/24 hrs.	Ochronosis, arthritis, spondylitis in adulthood. Urine darkens on exposure to air or alkali.	Homogenistic acid is a metabolite in degradation of tyrosine.

Aminoacidopathy	Abnormal Enzyme	Metabolic Disturbance

Defects of the Sulfur Amino Acid Metabolism

Homocystine

Cystathionine synthase deficiency B_6 responsive	Cystathionine synthase	Homocystine and methionine in blood and urine. Low cystine in plasma s-adenosylhomocystine, lanthionine and AICHR in urine.
Cystathionine synthase deficiency B_6 unresponsive	Same as above.	Same as above.
Homocystinuria with methylmaloniaciduria	N^5-methyltetrahydrofolate methyltransferase and (?) methylmaloryl-CoA isomerase deficiency	Excessive homocystine, methylmalonic acid and cystathionine in blood and urine, low plasma methionine.
Decreased methylenetetrahydro-folate reductase	Methylenetetrahydrofolate reductase	Homocystine in blood and urine but no increase in methionine.
Cystathionine	Cystathionase	Cystathionine in urine and trace in blood.

Treatment	Clinical Features	Comment
B$_6$ 250 to 400 mg/24 hrs.	Mental retardation in some. Habitus like Marfan's syndrome, dislocated lenses, telangiectasia, malar flush, thromboses of veins and arteries, ocular lesions, psychiatric disturbances.	Urinary cyanide nitroprusside test positive.
1.5 mg/kg/24 hrs protein restriction with 10 mg/kg/24 hrs methionine but large amounts of L-cystine and choline.	Same as above.	Same as above.
B$_{12}$ in large doses parentally may be beneficial in type with intestinal malabsorption.	Lethargy, failure to thrive, mental retardation, neurological abnormalities, may be asymptomatic form as well.	Defect in metabolic pathway where N^5-methyltetrahydrofolate acts as methyl donor in homocystine metabolism. Two types: (1) intestinal malabsorption of B$_{12}$ (2) impaired cellular metabolism of B$_{12}$
Folic acid	Schizophrenia, mild mental retardation, seizures, muscle weakness, may be normal.	Episodes of schizophrenia reported to respond to folic acid.
B$_6$ 200 to 400 mg/24 hrs corrects difficulty in most cases.	Probably benign trait but severe retardation and seizures have been reported.	A few cases are unresponsive to B$_6$ and may reflect coenzyme coupling defect.

Aminoacidopathy	Abnormal Enzyme	Metabolic Disturbance
Cystine	unknown (?) cystine reductase	Generalized aminoaciduria, no increased cystine in blood or urine.
Sulfite oxidase deficiency	Sulfite oxidase	Sulfacystine in urine.
β-mercaptolaceto-cystine deficiency	β-mercaptolaceto-cystine	Disulfide of β-mercaptolacetate and cystine in urine.
Glutathionuria	α-glutamyltranspepitase	Glutathione in urine and blood.

Defects of the Branched-Chain Amino Acids

Maple Syrup Urine Disease (MSUD)

Classic MSUD	Branched-chain keto-acid decarboxylase (activity <5% of normal)	Leucine, isoleucine and valine in blood and urine
Intermittent MSUD	Same as above (activity 10 to 20% of normal between episodes)	None except during attack when leucine, isoleucine and valine may be found in urine and blood.

Treatment	Clinical Features	Comment
Cystine poor diet, renal transplantation, D-penicillamine.	Cystine deposits in many organs, failure to thrive, Fanconi syndrome, vitamin D-resistant rickets, renal failure, corneal deposits.	Three forms: (1) infantile with renal disease in first decade; (2) juvenile with renal disease in second decade; and (3) adult without renal disease but with corneal deposits.
None.	Severe and progressive mental retardation, ectopic lens.	One case reported.
None.	Retardation, grand mal seizures in an adult; has been seen in two normals.	Positive cyanide nitroprusside in urine.
None.	Retardation in adult.	One case reported.
Dietary restriction of leucine, isoleucine and valine. Peritoneal dialysis for acute treatment in perinatal period.	Onset soon after birth, anorexia, failure to thrive, hypertonicity, seizures, mental retardation, vomiting, acidosis, coma, death in infancy.	Urine has odor of maple syrup.
0 to 1.5 mg/kg/24 hrs of protein during attacks, peritoneal dialysis in acute exacerbation.	Intermittent symptoms may occur during periods of illness, mild retardation in some patients.	Can be fatal during exacerbation when illness produces increased tissue catabolism, onset in early childhood.

Aminoacidopathy	Abnormal Enzyme	Metabolic Disturbance
Mild nonintermittent MSUD	Same as above (activity <25% of normal)	Leucine, isoleucine, and valine in blood and urine.
Thiamine responsive MSUD	Same as above (activity 20% of normal)	Leucine, isoleucine, and valine in blood and urine.
Hypervalinemia	Valine aminotransferase	Valine in blood and urine.
Isovalericacidemia	Isovaleryl CoA dehydrogenase	Isovaleric acid in urine and blood.
β-methylcrotonylglycine β-hydroxyisovalericaciduria	(?) β-methylcrotonyl CoA carboxylase	β-methylcrotonylglycine and β-hydroxyisovaleric acid increased in blood and urine.
Methylmalonicaciduria		
B$_{12}$ unresponsive	Methylmalonyl CoA carbonylmutase	Methylmalonic acid in blood and urine.
B$_{12}$ responsive	Normal enzyme in presence of coenzyme form of B$_{12}$ (? defect in B$_{12}$ coenzyme)	Same as above.

Treatment	Clinical Features	Comment
Dietary restriction of leucine, isoleucine and valine or low protein diet.	Moderate mental retardation.	Onset in later childhood. May have exacerbations during acute illnesses.
10 mg/24 hrs of thiamine.	Mild mental retardation.	Thiamine pyrophosphate acts as coenzyme in first step of oxidative carboxylation of leucine, isoleucine, and valine.
Diet low in valine, 100 to 200 mg/kg/24 hrs.	Vomiting, nystagmus, hyperkinesis, hypotonia, failure to thrive and mental retardation.	
Low protein diet with specific low leucine intake.	Mild mental retardation, episodes of acidosis and vomiting, lethargy and coma.	Urine has odor of sweaty feet; may have exacerbations during periods of intercurrent infection.
Two forms, one biotin responsive, other may respond to protein restriction particularly leucine.	Mental retardation, hypotonia, metabolic acidosis, vomiting, irritability.	Urine has odor of cat urine.
Diet low in protein (1.5 gm/kg/24 hrs).	Vomiting, lethargy, ketoacidosis, failure to thrive, mental retardation, death in infancy.	
B_{12} in large doses.	Same as above.	B_{12} to mother carrying affected fetus may be helpful.

Aminoacidopathy	Abnormal Enzyme	Metabolic Disturbance
Propionicaciduria		
Biotin unresponsive	Propionyl CoA carboxylase	Propionic acid in blood and urine.
Biotin responsive	Same as above.	Same as above.
Disorders of the Urea Cycle with Hyperammonemia		
Carbamylphosphate synthetase deficiency	Carbamylphosphate synthetase (CPS)	High blood ammonia glycine in blood and urine.
Ornithine transcarbamylase deficiency	Ornithine transcarbamylase	High blood ammonia glutamine in blood and urine, and orotic acid elevated in urine.
Hyperornithinemia	Unknown	High blood ammonia ornithine in blood and urine.
Citrullinemia	Argininosuccinic acid synthetase	High blood ammonia citrulline in blood and urine.
Argininosuccinicaciduria		
Neonatal type	Argininosuccinase	Argininosuccinic acid in blood and urine, high blood ammonia.
Subacute type	Same as above.	Same as above.

Treatment	Clinical Features	Comment
Protein restriction.	Recurrent attacks of ketoacidosis and neutropenia.	High protein intake or infections may precipitate attacks.
10 mg/24 hrs of biotin.	Same as above.	Same as above.
Low protein diet (1 gm/kg/24 hrs)	Episodic vomiting, lethargy, ketoacidosis, dehydration, seizures, mental retardation.	Absence of CPS activity in liver mitochondria.
Low protein diet (1.0 to 1.5 gm/kg/24 hrs)	Failure to thrive, vomiting, seizures, lethargy, coma, respiratory alkalosis, mental retardation.	Definite diagnosis made by assay of urea cycle enzymes in liver.
Low protein diet (1.5 gm/kg/24 hrs)	Irritability, vomiting, episodic abdominal pain, constipation.	
Low protein diet (1.0 to 1.6 gm/kg/24 hrs)	Vomiting, irritability, failure to thrive, mental retardation, seizures, ataxia.	
Low protein diet (1.4 to 1.6 gm/kg/24 hrs), exchange transfusion in acute state may be useful.	Lethargy, seizures, respiratory distress, friable hair.	All die in first two weeks.
Low protein diet (1.4 to 1.6 gm/kg/24 hrs)	Failure to thrive, mental retardation, hepatomegaly, friable hair.	Gradual onset.

Aminoacidopathy	Abnormal Enzyme	Metabolic Disturbance
Chronic type	Same as above.	Same as above.
Arginemia	Arginase	High blood ammonia, arginine in blood and urine, lysine, ornithine and cystine in urine.

Other Aminoacidopathies with Hyperammonemia

Hyperglycinemia

Ketotic form	Propionyl-CoA Carbon dioxide ligase	Glycine in blood and urine, high ammonia in blood.
Nonketotic form	(?) glycine decarboxylase	Glycine in blood and urine.

Hyperlysinemia

Persistent	Lysine α-ketoglutarate TPNH oxidoreductase	Lysine in blood and urine.
Nonpersistent	(?) partial defect of above	Lysine in blood and urine.
With saccharopinuria	(?) saccharopinase	Lysine, saccharopine and citrulline in blood and urine.

Treatment	Clinical Features	Comment
Same as above.	Intermittent ataxia, friable hair, psychomotor retardation, hepatomegaly.	Onset in second year of life.
Low protein diet (1.5 gm/kg/24 hrs)	Spastic diplegia, seizures, mental retardation.	
Low protein diet (0.5-1.5 gm/kg/24 hrs) oral electrolyte mixture may be needed in crisis.	Severe ketosis, lethargy, vomiting, coma, neutropenia, thrombocytopenia, myoclonic jerks.	
(?) low protein diet.	Severe mental retardation, seizures.	
Low protein diet (1.5-2.5 gm/kg/24 hrs) with low lysine (100 mg/kg/24 hrs)	Coma, vomiting, seizures, mental retardation, hypotonia.	
(?) same	Vomiting, seizures and episodic coma.	Episodes related to protein intake or infection.
(?) low protein	Mental retardation and short stature.	

Aminoacidopathy	Abnormal Enzyme	Metabolic Disturbance
Iminoacidopathies		
Hyperprolinemia		
Type I	Proline oxidase	Proline in blood and urine, hydroxyproline and glycine in urine.
Type II	Δ'-pyrioline-5-carboxylate dehydrogenase	Proline in blood and urine, Δ'-pyrioline-5-carboxylate, hydroxyproline and glycine in urine.
Hydroxyprolinemia	Hydroxyproline oxidase	Hydroxyproline in urine and blood
Other Aminoacidopathies		
Histidinemia	L-histidineammonialyase (Histadase)	Histadine in blood and urine, (?) alanine in blood and urine.
Hyper-β-alaninemia	(?) β-alanetransaminase	β-alanine, β-aminoisobutyric acid and taurine in blood and urine.
Carnosinemia	Carnosinase	Carosine in blood and urine
Hypersarcosinemia	Sarcosine oxygen oxidoreductase	Sarcosine in blood and urine.
Hartnup disease	Transport defect of neutral amino acids in kidney and intestine.	Neutral aminoacids in urine.

Treatment	Clinical Features	Comment
(?) low protein diet	Hereditary nephritis, seizures, deafness, mental retardation, may be normal.	May be benign.
(?) low protein diet	Mental retardation, seizures, may be normal.	May be benign.
(?) low protein diet	Mental retardation, psychotic behavior, may be normal.	May be benign.
(?) low protein diet	Speech defect, mental retardation, may be normal.	May be benign.
(?) large doses B_6	Somnolence, uncontrollable seizures, mental retardation.	
None known (?) zinc cofactor	Seizures, mental retardation.	
	Mental retardation, may be normal.	May be benign.
100 to 400 mg/24 hrs nicotinamide for rash.	Mental retardation, light sensitive rash, ataxia.	May be benign.

STORAGE AND DEGENERATIVE DISEASES OF THE CENTRAL NERVOUS SYSTEM[452, 453]

Disease	Enzyme Deficit	Inheritance	Age of Onset
Gaucher's disease (Cerebroside storage disease)			
Infantile (Type II)	β-glucosidase	autosomal recessive	Within the first year of life.
Juvenile (Type III)	β-glucosidase	autosomal recessive	1 to 5 years.
Adult (Type I)	β-glucosidase	autosomal recessive, may be some autosomal dominant forms.	30 to 40 years.
Niemann-Pick disease (Sphingomyeline Storage Disease)			
Group A (Type I) Classic acute infantile	sphingomyelinase	autosomal recessive	First year of life.

Neurological Signs and Symptoms	Nonneurological Signs and Symptoms	Comment
Progressive spasticity, progressive rigidity in opistatonic posture, autonomic nervous system dysfunction, strabismus, dysphagia, brain stem signs.	Failure to thrive, hepatosplenomegaly, enlarged lymphoid tissue, bone marrow infiltration producing anemia, thrombocytopenia and leukopenia.	80% mortality by one year; Gaucher cells in the bone marrow and viscera.
Borderline intelligence, seizures, stiffness, clumsiness, movement disorders, poor coordination, hyperactivity, eye movement difficulty	Hepatosplenomegaly, bone marrow involvement with anemia, thrombocytopenia and leukopenia, pathological fractures, Erlenmeyer flask deformities of bones.	Gaucher cells in viscera and bone marrow, death due to hematologic complications.
99% no central nervous system involvement.	Hepatosplenomegaly, hematological abnormalities secondary to bone marrow infiltration, pinguenculae of sclerae, yellow pigmentation of skin, orthopedic defects.	Long clinical course.
Regression in development, myoclonic jerks, exaggerated startle	Failure to thrive, hepatosplenomegaly, yellow discoloration of	50% Jewish ancestry; Neimann-Pick storage cells; progressive

Disease	Enzyme Deficit	Inheritance	Age of Onset
Group B (Type II) Heavy visceral and no CNS	sphingomyelinase	autosomal recessive	After first year of life.
Group C (Type III) Moderate visceral and little CNS	sphingomyelinase	autosomal recessive	Late childhood, early adult
Group D (Type IV) Nova Scotia variant	normal enzymes	autosomal recessive	Early childhood.
GM$_1$ gangliosidosis (general gangliosidosis)	ganglioside β-galactosidase	autosomal recessive	Symptoms from birth, by 8 months very apparent.

Neurological Signs and Symptoms	Nonneurological Signs and Symptoms	Comment
reflex, 40% cherry red macula, optic atrophy, deafness, seizures, brain stem signs, decerebrate posturing.	skin, bone marrow infiltration producing anemia, thrombocytopenia and leukopenia, demineralization of bone.	downhill course and death in early childhood.
None.	Hepatosplenomegaly, intermittent jaundice, bone marrow suppression.	There is an *adult form (Type E)*.
Emotional lability, cerebellar signs, dizziness, tremor, hyperactivity.	Hepatosplenomegaly, may have bone marrow suppression.	
Same as Group A.	Same as Group C.	Death in adolescence.

Cherry red spots 50%, macrocephaly may develop, regressive development, internal strabismus, poor suck, hypoactive DTRs, exaggerated startle response, seizures, terminal blindness and deafness, cytoplasmic membrane inclusion bodies on electron microscopic examination of neurons.	Poor appetite, weak suck, poor weight gain, peripheral edema, frontal bossing, depressed nasal bridge, low set ears, increased distance from nose to upper lip, downy hirsuitism, gum hypertrophy, macroglossia, hepatosplenomegaly, short broad hands and fingers, joint stiffness with contractures, hard nontender enlargement of wrist and ankle joints, hypoplastic beaked vertebral bodies, midshaft thickening of long bones, widening of ribs and flared ilium.	Dysmorphic features increase with time, death by 2 years. There is a *pure cerebral form without peripheral manifestations;* rectal biopsy may show deposition in neuronal cells and foamy cells may be seen in urine sediment.

Disease	Enzyme Deficit	Inheritance	Age of Onset
Amaurotic familial idiocy			
GM$_2$ gangliosidosis			
Infantile (Tay-Sachs)	unknown	autosomal recessive	1 to 4 years.
Juvenile	hexosaminidase A	autosomal recessive	3 to 6 years.
Sandhoff-Jatzekewitz	hexosaminidase A and B	autosomal recessive	4 to 6 months.
Ceroid lipofuscinoses			
Infantile (Trovey)	Unknown.	autosomal recessive	One year.

Neurological Signs and Symptoms	Nonneurological Signs and Symptoms	Comment
Withdrawn behavior, loss of interest in environment, incontinence, gradual psychomotor deterioration, optic atrophy and blindness, seizures early in disease, motor signs with increased tone and deep tendon reflexes.	None.	Death within the first 6 years.
Seizures, regression in development with intellectual deterioration, ataxia, increasing motor dysfunction, cherry red macula not seen	None.	Death usually in the first or second decade.
Same as Tay-Sachs.	Hepatosplenomegaly, long bone involvement, renal involvement; there may be secondary hematopoietic difficulties such as anemia, leukopenia, thrombocytopenia.	Death usually in the first decade.
Regression in development, retardation, ataxia, hypopigmentation of the retina, optic atrophy, seizures including myoclonic jerks, progressive motor deterioration and progressive cerebellar signs.	None.	Death in the end of the first decade.

Disease	Enzyme Deficit	Inheritance	Age of Onset
Jansky-Bielschowsky	Unknown.	autosomal recessive	1 to 4 years.
Batten Spielmeyer-Vogt-Sjögren	Unknown.	autosomal recessive	4 to 8 years.
Kufs'	Unknown.	autosomal recessive, some question of autosomal dominant inheritance	6 to 18 months.
Mucopoly-saccharidosis Hurler's (Type I)	α-iduronidase	autosomal recessive	6 to 18 months.

Neurological Signs and Symptoms	Nonneurological Signs and Symptoms	Comment
Seizures, optic atrophy, macular degeneration, progressive apathy and withdrawal from the environment and disinterest with a regression in development, early incontinence where child was previously continent, motor signs and movement disorders.	None.	Death in the first decade.
An early sign is regression in knowledge, change in personality, regression in speech patterns, visual loss becomes more prominent with time leading to blindness; there is retinal degeneration; seizures occur later in the disease; motor and cerebellar dysfunction.	Peripheral pigmentation occasionally occurs.	Death within the first or second decade.
Gradual loss of intellectual knowledge and change in personality, myoclonic seizures, cerebellar signs.		Long clinical course.
Macrocephaly, mental retardation, regressive development, hypotonia, corneal opacities, spasticity, deafness.	Coarse facial features including thickened lips, low nasal bridge, mild hypertelorism, prominent supraorbital ridges, diffuse nasal discharge, cardiomegaly with systolic murmur, prominent abdomen, hepatosplenomegaly,	Reilly bodies (metachromatic cytoplasmic inclusions) are found in 5% of peripheral lymphocytes, dermatin sulfate and heparatin sulfate found in the urine,

Disease	Enzyme Deficit	Inheritance	Age of Onset
Hunter's (Type II)	sulfoidurono-sulfatase	sex-linked recessive	2 to 4 years.
Sanfilippo's (Type III)	sulfatase α-n acetyl glucosaminidase	autosomal recessive	1 to 3 years.
Morquio's (Type IV)	sulfate cleaving enzyme from glucuronic acid	autosomal recessive	1 to 3 years.

Neurological Signs and Symptoms	Nonneurological Signs and Symptoms	Comment
	umbilical hernia, hypertrophied gums, gibbus, limitation of movement of joints, thickening of skin, kyphosis, flaring of the ribs, wedging of the vertebrae, short stubby fingers, clawlike deformity of the hand, hirsuitism.	deterioration and death usually in first decade.
No corneal cloudiness, otherwise similar to Hurler's.	Similar to Hurler's. No gibbus.	Dermatin sulfate and heparatin sulfate in the urine, slowly progressive course with death in the second to third decade.
Most severe retardation of the mucopolysaccharidoses, no corneal clouding, long course with gradual regression in development.	Mild shortness of stature, mild coarsening of facial features similar to Hurler's, mild joint immobility, thickening of the ribs, mild hirsuitism, mild hepatosplenomegaly.	Long course with very mild peripheral manifestations but with profound mental retardation. Individuals may live up to their fourth or fifth decade. Two different enzyme deficits, heparatin sulfate in urine.
Normal intelligence, hearing loss, corneal clouding.	Short neck, fusion of cervical vertebrae with platybasia, thoracic kyphosis, scoliosis, prominent sternum, flaring of ribs, widening of long bones with shortening of the long bones, lax joints, mild coarsening of facial features.	Keratosulfate secreted in urine, cardiac complications leading to death in second or third decade.

Disease	Enzyme Deficit	Inheritance	Age of Onset
Scheie's (Type V) (variant of Type I)	α-iduronidase	autosomal recessive	Childhood
Maroteaux-Lamy (Type VI)	sulfatide sulfatase	autosomal recessive	1 to 3 years.
β-glucuronidase deficiency (Type VII)	β-glucuronidase	autosomal recessive	1 to 3 years.
I-cell disease	sialidase	autosomal recessive	Infancy.
Oligosaccharidosis Manosidosis	α-manosidase	autosomal recessive	Infancy.
Fucosidosis	α-fucosidase	autosomal recessive	Infancy.

Neurological Signs and Symptoms	*Nonneurological Signs and Symptoms*	*Comment*
No or minimal impairment of intelligence, early corneal clouding, psychosis, regression in mental development may occur later in disease, hearing loss.	Coarsened facial features later in disease, limitation of joint motions later in disease with claw deformity of hand, hirsuitism, aortic valvular defect.	Dermaratin sulfate and heparatin sulfate in the urine.
Intelligence normal initially, possibly some mild mental regression later in life, corneal clouding.	Growth retardation, lumbar kyphosis, sternal protrusion, joint stiffness, widening of the long bones, wedging of the vertebrae, broadening of the ribs, genu valgum, hepatosplenomegaly, coarse facial features.	Dermaratin sulfate found in the urine.
Mild mental retardation.	Mild bony and facial changes.	
Similar to Hurler's disease, marked gibbus.	Similar to Hurler's disease.	Excess sialic acid in urine, defect in ability to incorporate enzymes into cell organelles.
Similar to Hurler's disease, no corneal cloudiness, deafness and unsteady gait are prominent.	Tremendously hypertrophied gums, otherwise similar to Hurler's disease.	Defect in the ability to form glycoprotein.
Similar to Hurler's disease, no corneal opacity, macrocephaly, severe mental retardation.	Similar to Hurler's disease.	Vacuoles found in lymphocytes and hepatic cells. There is an *adult form* where mental retardation occurs with a milder course and survival to old age.

Disease	Enzyme Deficit	Inheritance	Age of Onset
Aspartylglycos-aminuria	aspartynase	autosomal recessive	Infancy.
Xanthomatosis Farber's disease	ceramidase	autosomal recessive	Infancy.
Wolman's disease	acid lipase	autosomal recessive	Early infancy.
Cerebrotendonis xanthomatosis (cholesterol storage disease)	cholesterol synthetase	presumed autosomal recessive	Adolescence.
Sulphatide Leukodystrophy (Metachromatic leukodystrophy) Type I Juvenile	sulfatide sulfatase	autosomal recessive	1 to 6 years.

Neurological Signs and Symptoms	Nonneurological Signs and Symptoms	Comment
Similar to Hurler's disease.	Similar to Hurler's disease.	Scandinavian heritage, live into late childhood.
Hypertonia, mental retardation, hoarseness of voice.	Failure to thrive, constriction of joint movement, swelling of joints especially in the fingers, subcutaneous nodules.	Death within the first 1 to 2 years, may be a *variant with late onset* and no CNS involvement.
Delay in development.	Large calcified adrenals, failure to thrive, hepatosplenomegaly, bone marrow infiltration with secondary anemia and thrombocytopenia, foam cells found in the adrenals, bone marrow, liver, and spleen.	Death by 3 to 4 months. There may be an *adult variant.*
Cerebellar signs with ataxia.	Thickened tendons secondary to cholesterol deposits.	Cholesterol deposits in the brain stem, cerebellum, and dentate nucleus.
Regression in motor skills, regression in intellectual performance, unsteadiness, diminution in deep tendon reflexes, nystagmus, speech becomes dysarthric, loss of bladder control, episodes of hyperpyrexia, blindness and deafness, elevation in cerebrospinal fluid protein.	Involvement of the gallbladder with gallstone production, involvement of kidney cells leading to metachromatic material in urine sediment, involvement of the islets of Langerhans of the pancreas, occasionally lymph node and adrenal involvement.	Metachromasia refers to change in color of the stored material in cells so that dyes that usually stain blue take on a red-brown color. There is involvement of the peripheral nerves so that there is a delayed nerve conduction velocity. Stored material may be demonstrated on nerve biopsy. Death within the first decade.

Disease	Enzyme Deficit	Inheritance	Age of Onset
Type II Adult	sulfatide sulfatidase	autosomal recessive, may be some autosomal dominant forms.	30 years.
Miscellaneous Fabry's disease	α-galactosidase	sex-linked recessive	Childhood.
Refsum's disease	phytanic acid α-hydroxatase	autosomal recessive	Childhood.
Krabbe's (globoid cell leukodystrophy)	cerebroside β-galactosidase	autosomal recessive	Infancy.

Neurological Signs and Symptoms	Nonneurological Signs and Symptoms	Comment
Slowly progressive spasticity and ataxia, psychological difficulties.	Same as juvenile form.	Long, slowly progressive course.
Episodic indescribable incapacitating pain initially involving fingers and toes, mild mental retardation, seizures, deposition of stored material in peripheral neurons in sympathetic and other plexuses, corneal deposits and strokes.	Peripheral manifestations red to purple macules and papules called angiokeratoma, fine telangiectasia, renal disease with polyuria and diabetes insipidus, also progressive renal hypertension, deposition of lipid deposits in the blood vessels.	Death secondary to renal complications or stroke, renal transplantation will reverse symptomatology.
Retinal pigment with constriction of visual fields, progressive polyneuropathy, increased CSF protein, nystagmus, deafness, ataxia, night blindness, steppage gait, anosmia.	Icthiosis.	Dietary restriction of phytanic acid may be helpful in halting progression, palpable thickening of peripheral nerves are present, no change in mentation.
Hypertonicity, optic atrophy, spasticity, increased deep tendon reflexes, blindness, hyperacousis, temperature instability, peripheral neuropathy present with involvement of peripheral neuronal plexuses, macrocephaly.	Failure to thrive.	Death usually in first two years. Neuropathological hallmarks are globoid cells in the white matter. There may be some atypical cases with delayed onset in late infancy and early childhood.

Disease	Enzyme Deficit	Inheritance	Age of Onset
Alexander's disease	Unknown	presumed autosomal recessive	Infancy.
Canavan's disease (diffuse spongy sclerosis)	Unknown.	autosomal recessive	Early infancy.
Pelizaeus-Merzbacker	Unknown.	sex-linked recessive	Infancy.
Cockayne's syndrome	Unknown.	autosomal recessive	First year of life.
Schilder's disease (adrenoleuko-dystrophy)	Unknown.	sex-linked recessive	Childhood.

Neurological Signs and Symptoms	Nonneurological Signs and Symptoms	Comment
Regression in development, seizures, spastic quadriplegia, atrophy of muscles, megencephaly.	None	Neuropathological hallmarks are eosinophilic deposits especially around the blood vessels. (Rosenthal fibers).
Marked mental retardation, hypotonia progressing to hypertonia, involuntary movements, optic atrophy, macrocephaly.	None.	Neuropathological hallmark is involvement of U-fibers of the white matter with a spongy form of encephalopathy.
Initial rapid progression with seizures, eye rolling, twitching, mental retardation, microcephaly, pallor of the optic discs, nystagmus, uncoordinated limb movements and ataxia. The patient then has a slowly progressive deterioration.	None.	Death usually in the second decade. Neuropathological hallmark is a tigroid appearance to white matter with fat stain. There are some variants of this disease with variable ages of onset.
Severe mental retardation, optic atrophy, deafness, slowly progressive course, ataxia, tremor, retinal pigmentation.	Prognathism, thickening of skull bones, kyphoscoliosis, cold blue limbs, beaked nose, large ears.	Death in the third to fourth decade, may be a variant of Pelizaeus-Merzbacker disease.
Spasticity, progressive cortical blindness, progressive deafness, optic atrophy, progressive dementia.	Adrenal failure secondary to deposition of cholesterol in the adrenal gland, brownish discoloration of the skin.	There appears to be a *nonsex-linked recessive form without adrenal involvement* and without brownish discoloration of skin.

Disease	Enzyme Deficit	Inheritance	Age of Onset
Lafora's body disease (Unverricht's disease)	Unknown.	autosomal recessive	7 to 14 years.
Lesch-Nyhan disease	hypoxanthine quanine phosphoribosyl transferase	sex-linked recessive	Early childhood.
Hallervorden-Spatz disease	Unknown.	presumed autosomal recessive	Late childhood.
Galactosemia	galactose 1-phosphate uridyl transeferase	autosomal recessive	Early infancy.
Menke's kinky hair disease	Unknown.	sex-linked recessive	Early infancy.

Neurological Signs and Symptoms	Nonneurological Signs and Symptoms	Comment
Seizures, massive myoclonic jerks, ataxia, choreoathetosis, dementia, cerebellar signs, retinal changes. In the end stages the seizures are refractory to all anticonvulsant medications and become constant within 10 years of onset.	Lafora bodies have been found in heart and liver.	Neuropathological hallmark are intercytoplasmic inclusion bodies in the neurons (Lafora bodies). The massive myoclonic jerks seen in this disease may become incapacitating. The course is very slowly progressive.
Progressive mental retardation, choreoathetosis, seizures, spasticity, self mutilation.	Hyperuricemia, gouty tophi, elevated uric acid in the serum, late onset renal disease secondary to uric acid crystals and stones.	Patients will self mutilate fingers, toes and lips; self mutilation becomes progressively worse with time.
Progressive movement disorder with dystonia or choreoathetosis, rigidity which is also progressive.	None.	There is deposition of iron containing pigment in the basal ganglia neuropathologically.
Mental retardation, cataracts.	Hepatosplenomegaly, cirrhosis, nausea, vomiting, generalized aminoaciduria.	Treatment is possible by the elimination of galactose from the diet starting early in infancy. Early treatment will prevent mental retardation.
Progressive psychomotor deterioration, severe seizures, optic atrophy, hypertonia, irritability.	Twisted early friable hair which has a steel wool-like quality, anemia, feeding difficulties, small for gestational age.	The disease is secondary to a defect in copper metabolism and copper absorption from the intestine. Death within the first 3 years.

Disease	Enzyme Deficit	Inheritance	Age of Onset
Wilson's disease (hepatolenticular degeneration)	Unknown.	autosomal recessive	Late childhood to early adolescence.
Huntington's disease (juvenile form)	Unknown.	autosomal dominant	Early childhood.
Leigh's disease (subacute necrotizing encephalo-myelopathy)	thiamine inhibitor	autosomal recessive	Variable throughout childhood but usually early childhood.

Neurological Signs and Symptoms	Nonneurological Signs and Symptoms	Comment
Tremor, gait disturbance, speech disturbance, progressive dementia, psychiatric difficulties, Kayser-Fleischer ring in the cornea.	Cirrhosis and hepatitis, anemia, leukopenia and thrombocytopenia, bluish discoloration of the fingernail beds.	This condition is secondary to a defect in copper metabolism where there is a partial lack in ceruloplasm, the copper carrying protein of the blood. Neurological signs and symptoms may be improved by the addition of a low copper diet and enhanced renal secretion of copper.
Regression in performance and development, hyperactivity, temper tantrums, clumsiness, slurring of speech, chorioform movements. With time these symptoms worsen. Rigidity, bradykinesia and Parkinsonianlike gait appears.	None.	This is a progressive degenerative disease leading to death within the first to second decade.
The disease is characterized by remissions and relapses, seizures, hypotonia, eye movement abnormalities, cranial nerve palsies, optic atrophy, spasticity, breathing difficulties on a central basis, mental retardation.	Failure to thrive.	The clinical course of this disease is highly variable. The duration of the illness is from a few weeks to several years.

Appendix C

OTHER GENETIC AND CHROMOSOMAL DISORDERS[72, 160, 161, 454]

Disease	Inheritance	Craniofacial Malformation
Chromosomal Syndrome		
Trisomy 21 (Down's syndrome, mongolism)	full trisomy 21 or DG or GG translocations	Brachycephalic, flattened facies, small nose, upward slant to palpebral fissures, epicanthal folds, Brushfield spots in iris, lens opacities, hypoplastic teeth.
Trisomy 18	18 trisomy	Prominent occiput, scaphiocephalic head, low set ears, micrognathia, narrow high arched palate, microcephaly may occur, cleft hip and/or palate may occur.
Trisomy 13	13 trisomy	Microcephaly, microphthalmia, coloboma of iris, retinal dysplasia, cleft lip and/or palate, abnormal ears, holoprosencephaly either partial or complete, multiple possible abnormalities of brain fusion and cleavage, hypotelorism of varying degrees including cyclopia, anophthalamus may occur, micrognathia may occur.

Skeletal Malformations	*Other Malformations*	*Comment*
Short stubby fingers, clinodactyly of fifth finger, wide gap between first and second toes, hypoplastic pelvis with shallow acetabular angle and flaring of the iliac crest.	Endocardial cushing defects, fine soft sparse hair, simian crease, widened palmar axial triradial angle, abnormal sternal loop pattern on all digits.	Hypotonia usually most marked in the neonatal and infantile periods, mental deficiency in all cases, seizures may occur, presenile dementia common.
Overlapping of index, third and fifth fingers over the fourth finger, short sternum, small pelvis, rockerbottom feet may occur.	Abnormal dermal ridge pattern, hypoplastic nails, inguinal and umbilical hernia, cardiac anomalies.	Small for gestational age, mental retardation, spasticity.
Finger flexion with overlapping digits, polydactyly, prominent calcanias, hypoplastic pelvis with abnormal acetabular angle.	Abnormal palmar axial triradial angle, simian crease, hyperconvex fingernails, cardiac anomalies, abnormal genitalia, inguinal or umbilical hernias, single umbilical artery in cord.	Minor motor seizures including massive infantile spasms may occur, severe mental retardation, deafness is common.

Disease	Inheritance	Craniofacial Malformation
Deletion of chromosome #4	4p-	Fish-like mouth, epicanthal folds, cleft lip and/or palate, strabismus, deformity of iris, hypotelorism, broad beaked nose, microcephaly, preauricular dimple, low set ears, may have midline scalp defect.
Cri du chat syndrome	5p-	Microcephaly, antimongoloid slant of eyes, hypertelorism, epicanthal folds, strabismus, rounded face, low set malformed ears, cleft lip and/or palate.
Deletion of long arm of chromosome 18	18q-	Midfacial hypoplasia, microcephaly, deep set eyes, carplike mouth, narrow palate, ear abnormalities, may have epicanthal fold and other eye anomalies.
Deletion of short arm of chromosome 18	18p-	Epicanthal folds, ptosis, saddle nose, carplike mouth, abnormal ears, may have other eye anomalies and facial clefts.
Deletion of long arm of 21	21q-	Antimongoloid slant, redundant skin over eyelids, micrognathia, wide malformed ears.

Skeletal Malformations	Other Malformations	Comment
May have delayed boneage, growth deficiency.	Hypoplastic dermal ridges, simian creases, genital abnormalities, small for gestational age with continued delayed growth.	Seizures and severe mental retardation are common.
	Simian crease, abnormal axial triradial angle, congenital heart disease.	Hypotonia and severe mental retardation are common, characteristic feature is a catlike cry in infancy, small for gestational age with slow growth during life.
Long hands with tapering fingers, abnormal toes, equinovarus deformity of foot.	Cardiac defects, skin dimples over knuckles, genital abnormalities, abnormal digital whirl pattern, simian creases, abnormal axial triradial angles.	Mental deficiency, hypotonia common, deafness, nystagmus, and poor coordination are also seen.
Short stature, minor anomalies of fingers and toes.	Failure to thrive.	Mental retardation and hypotonia are common, females affected greater than males, clinical stigmata are not characteristic in all cases, verbal development more affected than motor.
Retarded bone maturation.	Dysplastic nails, abnormal axial triradial angle, hypogonadism, thrombocytopenia, pyloric stenosis.	Small for testational age, increased tone and mental deficiency in all cases.

Disease	Inheritance	Craniofacial Malformation
Ring chromosome #18	18 ring	Round face, hypertelorism, epicanthal folds, ear anomalies, flat occiput.
Tetra X/Y (Klinefelter's syndrome)	XXXXY	Antimongoloid eyes, epicanthal folds, strabismus, prognathism, abnormal ears, flattened nasal bridge with retrousse nose, wide set eyes.
Penta X	XXXXX	Mongoloid slant to eyes.
Turner's syndrome	XO	Small mandible, narrow slightly high arched palate, mild antimongoloid slant to eyes, epicanthal folds may be seen.
Noonan's syndrome (male Turner's)	unknown	Epicanthal folds, low set malformed ears.

Neurocutaneous Syndromes

Neurofibromatosis (von Recklinghausen's disease)	autosomal dominant with high mutation rate	

Skeletal Malformations	*Other Malformations*	*Comment*
Short stature, club foot, cindactyly.		Mental retardation, microcephaly, and deafness may occur.
Fifth finger clindactyly, synostosis of radius and ulna, pes planus.	Short stature, delayed bone maturation, short neck, abnormal ridge count on fingertips, hypoplastic genitalia, small for gestational age.	Mental deficiency in all cases, limited elbow pronation, hypotonia, joint laxity.
Small hand, clindactyly of fifth finger	Patent ductus arteriosus.	Severe mental deficiency, growth deficiency, may be small for gestational age.
Broad chest with widely spaced nipples, pectus excavatum, elbow anomalies, knee anomalies, short fourth toe, dysplastic bone.	Short stature, varying agensis, short webbed neck with low posterior hairline, fingernail anomalies, cardiac defect may occur primarily coarctation of the aorta.	May have hearing impairment but intelligence is normal.
Pectus excavatum, shieldlike chest, vertebral column anomalies.	Short stature, webbed neck with low posterior hairline, congenital heart disease primarily pulmonic stenosis, hypoplastic genitalia.	Mental retardation in most cases, no known chromosomal abnormality but phenotypically resembles Turner's. Not true chromosome disorder.

Neurocutaneous Syndromes

Scoliosis, bone cysts, pseudoarthoses, asymmetrical bone overgrowth, vertebral anomalies.	Multiple areas of café au lait spots, subcutaneous tumors of the nerve sheaths, plexiform neuromas, neurofibromas may involve other organs such as kidneys and heart.	Subcutaneous tumors may undergo malignant change, increased incidence of brain neoplasms, mental retardation or seizures may occur.

Disease	Inheritance	Craniofacial Malformation
Tuberosclerosis (adenoma sebacium)	autosomal dominant with high spontaneous mutation rate.	Hemartomatous lesions in brain substance and in retina. These lesions may calcify; development of fibrous angiomatous lesions in butterfly distributions over face.
Sturge-Weber syndrome	suspect autosomal dominant with high spontaneous mutation rate	Red-purple cutaneous flat hemangiomata over the face in distribution of the trigeminal nerve usually involving one or more divisions on the same side of the face, glaucoma and exophthalmos may occur; there is involvement of the ipsilateral, occipital parietal or temporal areas with hemangiomata involving the arachnoid and pia; cortical atrophy and calcification occurs in the cortical convolutions.
Von Hippel-Lindau syndrome	autosomal dominant with varying expressivity	Angioma of the retina, cerebellar angiomatous tumors, occasionally hemangioblastomas with cysts.
Ataxia telangiectasia (Louis-Bar syndrome)	autosomal dominant	Progressive cerebellar hypoplasia, telangiectasia of bulbar conjunctiva, also ear and neck may be involved.

Skeletal Malformations	Other Malformations	Comment
Bone cysts in phalanges.	Café au lait spots, areas of hypopigmentation, subungal fibromas, chagrin patches.	Seizures are exceptionally common in infancy. They may be manifested as massive infantile spasms; high incidence of mental retardation, increased incidence of central nervous system and peripheral neoplasms. such as kidney, heart, liver, and pancreas.
	Hemangiomata may be seen in other areas of the body.	Seizures are common; contralateral hemiparesis is frequently seen; most patients are mentally deficient.
	Hemangiomata may occur in other parts of body including face, kidney, pancreas, and liver. There may be associated cysts of pancreas, liver and kidney.	With advancing age, cerebellar dysfunction becomes more apparent.
	Occurrence of sino-pulmonary infections, decreased IgA, paucity of lymphoid tissue, high incidence of malignancies	Ataxia usually begins in the second year and becomes progressively worse, choreoathetosis may

Disease	Inheritance	Craniofacial Malformation

Syndromes of Craniofacial Dysostosis

Disease	Inheritance	Craniofacial Malformation
Crouzon's disease	autosomal dominant variable expressivity	Premature craniosynostosis, facial bone abnormalities, shallow orbits with oculoproptosis, hypertelorism hypoplastic mandible, beak-like nose.
Carpenter's syndrome	suspect autosomal recessive	Premature craniosynostosis, acrocephaly, lateral displacement of inner canthi facial bone abnormalities.
Apert's syndrome	autosomal dominant with high mutation rate	Cranial synostosis, midfacial hypoplasia with facial bone abnormalities, flat face, shallow orbits, antimongoloid slant to eyes, small beaking nose and maxillary hypoplasi midline palatal defects may be seen.

Other Syndromes

Disease	Inheritance	Craniofacial Malformation
Treacher-Collins syndrome	autosomal dominant with high spontaneous mutation rate	Antimongoloid slant to eyes mandibular hypoplasia, coloboma of lower lid, malformed ears and ear canals, microthalmia and cleft palate may occur.
Goldenhar's syndrome	suspect autosomal recessive	Lipomas of the conjunctiva cleft of upper eyelid, malformed ears, hypoplasti xygomatic arches, mandibul hypoplasia, malar hypoplasi dental maloeclusions.

Skeletal Malformations	Other Malformations	Comment
	especially of the lymphoreticular system, increased sedimentation rate, insulin-resistant diabetes.	occur, retardation may occur.
		Surgical correction of cranial synostosis is purely cosmetic. Some individuals may have developmental disabilities.
Polydactyly and syndactyly may occur.	Hypoplastic genitalia, obesity.	Mental retardation is characteristic.
Syndactyly of fingers and toes, shortening of fingers and toes.		High incidence of mental retardation but normal intelligence may occur.
Vertebral anomalies may occur.	Congenital heart defects may occur.	Mental retardation may occur.
Vertebral anomalies may occur.		Mental retardation may occur; deafness is often seen.

Disease	Inheritance	Craniofacial Malformation
Cornelia de Lange syndrome	Unknown.	Microcephaly, brachycephaly, synorphism, long thick eye lashes, small retrousse nose, high arched palate, carp-like mouth, micrognathia.
Rubinstein-Taybi syndrome	sporadic occurrence	Antimongoloid slant of eyes, beaked nose with nasal septum prominent, epicanthal folds, low set and/or malformed ears.
Prader-Willi syndrome	Unknown.	Strabismus.
Laurence-Moon-Biedle syndrome	suspect autosomal recessive	Retinitis pigmentosa.
Beckwith-Wiedemann syndrome	suspect autosomal recessive	Macroglossia, prominent metopic ridge on forehead, prominent occiput, mandibular prognathism, malformation of ears.
Soto's syndrome (cerebral gigantism)	unknown	Large cranium, prognathism coarse facies with full lips.
Smith-Lemli-Opitz syndrome	suspect autosomal recessive	Microcephaly, scaphocephaly malformed ears or low set ears, ptosis of eyelids, epicanthal folds, broad nasal bridge with retrousse nose, micrognathia.

Skeletal Malformations	Other Malformations	Comment
Short stature, delayed bone maturation, small hands and feet, clinodactyly of fifth finger, clinodactyly of toes, proximal implantation of thumb.	Hypoplastic genitalia, flexion contracture of elbow, simian crease, hypoplastic nipples.	Mental retardation in all cases, low pitched weak cry, small for gestational age.
Delayed bone maturation, broad thumbs and broad toes, short stubby fingers may occur, abnormal acetabular angle, flared ilium.	Short stature.	Borderline retardation in most cases.
Small hands and feet.	Small stature, obesity, hypoplastic genitalia, abnormal glucose tolerance.	Hypotonia and mental retardation.
Polydactyly and/or syndactyly.	Obesity, genital hypoplasia.	Mental retardation in most cases, renal defects and nerve deafness are common.
	Macrosomia, hyperplastic kidneys, hyperplastic pancreas, hyperplastic gonads, hyperplastic adrenal cortex, umphalocele or umbilical anomaly.	Hypoglycemia occurs in infancy, mental retardation is common.
Large hands, large feet, advanced bone maturation.	Thick subcutaneous tissue, excessive size throughout life, large for gestational age.	Borderline to retarded intellectual performance, poor coordination, seizures.
	Simian crease, hypogonadism and cryporchism in males, abnormal digital whirl pattern, small for gestational age.	Retardation of varying degrees, alterations of muscle tone noted.

Disease	Inheritance	Craniofacial Malformation
Riley-Day syndrome (familial dysautonomia)	suspect autosomal recessive common in Jewish people.	
William's syndrome	Unknown.	Broad wide mouth with broadened maxilla, retrousse small nose, hypertelorism, epicanthal folds, small mandible, prominent ears.
Donohue's syndrome (leprechaunism)	suspect autosomal recessive	Small prominent eyes, thick lips, large prominent ears, wide nostrils.
Lowe's syndrome (oculo-cerebro-renal syndrome)	sex-linked recessive	Cataracts, glaucoma.
Zellweger's syndrome (cerebro-hepato-renal syndrome)	presumed autosomal recessive	High forehead, epicanthal folds, flattened facies, mild mongoloid slant, macrogyria, polymicrogyria of the cortex.
Incontinentia pigmenti	autosomal or sex-linked recessive	Microcephaly, strabismus, retinal dysplasia, cataracts, blue sclerae, uvitis, keratitis, patchy alopoecia.

Skeletal Malformations	*Other Malformations*	*Comment*
Small stature, scoliosis is common.	Malfunction of the autonomic nervous system is the hallmark of this condition, consists of vomiting, diarrhea, lack of tearing, insensitivity To pain, skin blotching, taste difficulties, temperature instability, unstable blood pressure, absent deep tendon reflexes, poor coordination.	Mental deficiency and seizures often occur.
Osteosclerosis, hypoplastic teeth.	Supravalvular aortic stenosis common, may also have peripheral pulmonary artery stenosis.	Short stature common, small for gestational age, hypercalcemia in infancy, mental retardation.
Delayed bone maturation.	Hyperplastic genitalia, hirsuitism, iron deposition in liver, hypoglycemia may occur, marked lack of adipose tissue.	Retardation and motor deficits.
Osteoporosis and occasionally rickets.	Renal tubular dysfunction, cryptorchism.	Hyperactivity, mental retardation, hypotonia, joint hypermobility, absent deep tendon reflexes.
	Hepatomegaly, albuminuria, renal cysts, patent ductus arteriosus, cardiac septal defects.	Hypotonia, retardation, growth deficiency, excessive iron storage in this syndrome.
Syndactyly, hemiatrophy, vertebral and rib anomalies, hypodontia.	Atrophy and irregular grey brown pigmentation of the skin in whirl-like patterns.	Mental retardation, spasticity and seizures are common. A form of characteristic pigmentary

Disease	*Inheritance*	*Craniofacial Malformation*
Sjögren-Larsson syndrome	autosomal recessive, common in Swedish ancestry	Pigmentary retinal degeneration may occur; hypertelorism may occur.
Marinesco-Sjögren's syndrome	autosomal recessive	Cataracts, nystagmus, and dysarthria.

Syndromes of Altered Fetal Environment

Rubella	secondary to intrauterine exposure to Rubella virus in the first trimester	Microcephaly, cataracts, glaucoma, corneal opacities, chorioretinitis.
Fetal alcohol syndrome	secondary to exposure to large amounts of alcohol during gestation	Microcephaly, microscopic brain anomalies, short palpebral fissures, maxillary hypoplasia, epicanthal folds, micrognathia, cleft palate, carp-shaped mouth, hypoplastic nasal bridge, retrousse nose.
Fetal hydantoin syndrome	exposure to phenytoin during gestation	Hypertelorism, epicanthal folds, ptosis of eyelids, strabismus, short nose with flattened nasal bridge,

Skeletal Malformations	Other Malformations	Comment
		changes are present in early infancy but evolve into the characteristic adult pattern.
Short stature, hypoplasia of teeth and kyphosis.	Icthiosis, diminished sweating.	Mental retardation is characteristic; spasticity primarily in lower extremities is also characteristic.
Kyphoscoliosis may be seen.	Mild to moderate growth deficiency.	Cerebellar ataxia and hypotonia and mental retardation are consistent findings.
Osteolitic lesions of bone.	Growth deficiency, patent ductus arteriosus, peripheral pulmonic stenosis, cardiac septal defects, hepatosplenomegaly, obstructive jaundice, thrombocytopenia, and anemia in newborn period.	Deafness, seizures and retardation.
Joint anomalies, phalangeal anomalies.	Small for gestational age, postnatal growth deficiency, altered palmar creases, cardiac anomalies, genital anomalies, neural tube defects, renal anomalies.	Developmental delays are common with mild to moderate retardation.
fingerlike thumb, b, sternal or spinal anomalies, hypoplasia of distal phalanges.	Hypoplasia of nails, abnormal palmar crease, abnormal digital markings, short webbed neck with a	Mental retardation and motor dysfunction.

Disease	Inheritance	Craniofacial Malformation
		low set of abnormal ears, wide mouth, prominent lips, microcephaly, cleft palate may occur.

Skeletal Malformations	*Other Malformations*	*Comment*
	low hairline, coarse hair, hypoplastic nipples, cardiac defects may occur.	

BIBLIOGRAPHY

1. Kinsbourne, M.: School problems. *Pediatrics, 52:*697, 1973.
2. Illingworth, R. S.: *The Development of the Infant and Young Child: Normal and Abnormal,* 7th ed. Edinburgh, Livingstone, 1980.
3. Gesell, Arnold and Amatruda, Catherine S.: *Developmental Diagnosis: Normal and Abnormal Child Development,* 2nd ed. New York, Hoeber, 1957.
4. Sparrow, S. and Zigler, E.: Evaluation of a patterning treatment for retarded children. *Pediatrics, 62:*137, 1978.
5. Piper, M. C. and Pless, I. B.: Early intervention for infants with Down syndrome: A control trial. *Pediatrics, 65:*463, 1980.
6. MacKeith, R. C.: The placing response and primary walking. *Guy's Hospital Gazette, 79:*394, 1965.
7. Buda, F. B.: unpublished observation.
8. Twitchell, T. E.: The automatic grasping responses of infants. *Neuropsychology, 3:*247, 1965.
9. Rabe, E. F.: Neurological evaluation in minimal brain dysfunction in children. *Public Health Service Publication, 2015:*69, 1969.
10. Twitchell, T. E.: Minimal cerebral dysfunction in children: Motor defects. *Transactions of the American Medical Association, 91:*353, 1966.
11. McKay, I. A. W.: Strategies for clumsy children. *Dev Med Child Neurol, 20:*494, 1978.
12. Kinsbourne, M.: Minimal brain dysfunction as a neurodevelopmental lag. *Ann NY Acad Sci, 205:*268, 1973.
13. Travis, L. E.: *Handbook of Speech Pathology and Audiology.* New York, Appleton-Century-Crofts, 1971.
14. Rutter, M. and Martin, J. A. M.: *The Child with Delayed Speech: Clinics in Developmental Medicine #43.* Philadelphia, Lippincott, 1972.
15. Chall, J.: *Learning to Read: The Great Debate.* New York, McGraw-Hill, 1967.
16. Thompson, I. J.: Learning disabilities: An overview. *Am J Psychiatry, 130:*393, 1973.
17. Kinsbourne, M. and Warrington, E. K.: Developmental factors in reading and writing backwardness. *Br J Psychology, 54:*145, 1963.
18. Schmitt, B. D. et al.: The hyperactive child. *Clin Pediatr, 12:*154, 1973.
19. Cromwell, R. L., Palk, B. E. and Foshee, J. G.: Studies in activity level V: The relationships among eyelid conditioning, intelligence, activity level and age. *Am J Ment Defic, 65:*744, 1961.
20. Pick, A. D., Frankel, D. O., and Valerie, L. H.: Children's attention: The

development of selectivity. In Hetherington, I. M. (Ed.): *Review of Child Development Research.* Chicago, University of Chicago Press, 1975, vol. V.

21. Gilmore, J. V.: *Gilmore Oral Reading Test.* New York, Harcourt Brace & World, 1957.

22. Paine, R. S. and Oppe, T. E.: *The Neurological Examination of Children.* London, Em. Heinemann, 1966.

23. Livingstone, S.: *Comprehensive Management of Epilepsy in Infancy, Childhood and Adolescence.* Springfield, Thomas, 1972.

24. Walsh, F. B. and Hoyt, U. F.: *Clinical Neuro-Ophthalmology,* 3rd ed. Baltimore, Williams & Wilkins, 1969.

25. Cogan, D. G.: *Neurology of the Ocular Muscles,* 2nd ed. Springfield, Thomas, 1956.

26. Goss, C. M. (Ed.): *Gray's Anatomy of the Human Body,* 27th ed. Philadelphia, Lea & Febiger, 1959.

27. Crowley, H. and Kaufman, R. S.: The Rinne tuning fork test. *Arch Otolaryngol, 84:*406, 1966.

28. Glorig, A. (Ed.): *Audiometry: Principles and Practices.* Baltimore, Williams & Wilkins, 1965.

29. Swaiman, K. F. and Wright, F. S.: *Neuromuscular Diseases in Infancy and Childhood.* Springfield, Thomas, 1970.

30. Parr, C., Routh, D. K., and McMillan J.: A developmental study of the asymmetrical tonic neck reflex. *Dev Med Child Neurol, 16:*329, 1974.

31. Paine, R. S.: Neurologic examination of infants and children. *Pediatr Clin North Am, 7:*41, 1960.

32. Paine, R. S.: The evaluation of infantile postural reflexes in the presence of chronic brain syndromes. *Dev Med Child Neurol, 6:*345, 1964.

33. Paimelee, A. H., Jr.: A critical evaluation of the Moro reflex. *Pediatrics, 33:*773, 1964.

34. Twitchell, T. E.: The neurological examination in infantile cerebral palsy. *Dev Med Child Neurol, 5:*271, 1963.

35. Critchley, E. M.: The neurological examination of neonates. *J Neurol Sci, 7:*127, 1968.

36. Paine, R. S.: Neurologic conditions in the neonatal period: Diagnosis and management. *Pediatr Clin North Am, 8:*577, 1961.

37. Hogan, G. R. and Milligan, J. E.: The plantar reflex of the newborn. *New Engl J Med, 285:*502, 1971.

38. Denny-Brown, D.: *Handbook of Neurological Examination and Care Recording,* 2nd ed. Cambridge, Harvard University Press, 1957.

39. Twitchell, T. E.: The grasping deficit in infantile spastic hemiparesis. *Neurology (Minneap.), 8:*13, 1958.

40. DeJong, R. N.: Care taking and the neurological examination. In Baker, A. B. and Baker, L. H. (Eds.): *Clinical Neurology.* New York, Hayes & Row, 1977, vol. I, pp. 1-23.

41. Tax, H. R.: Pedopediatrics. In Weinstein, F. (Ed.): *Principles and Practice of Podiatry.* Philadelphia, Lea & Febiger, 1968, pp. 248-263.
42. Nellhaus, G.: Composite international and interracial graphs. *Pediatrics, 41:*106, 1968.
43. Popich, G. A. and Smith, D. W.: Fontanels: Range of normal size. *J Pediatr, 80:*749, 1972.
44. Dodge, P. R. and Porter, P.: Demonstration of intracranial pathology by transillumination. *Arch Neurol, 5:*594, 1961.
45. Childelin, L. V., Davis, P. C., and Grant, W. N.: Normal values for transillumination of skull using a new light source. *J Pediatr, 86:*937, 1975.
46. Langeman, J.: *Medical Embryology.* Baltimore, Williams & Wilkins, 1963, pp. 246-279.
47. Dulos, R., Savage, D., and Schaedler, R.: Biological Freudianism: Lasting effects of early environmental influences. *Pediatrics, 38:*789, 1966.
48. Davidson, A. N. and Dobbing, J.: *Applied Neurochemistry.* Oxford, Blackwell Scientific Publications, 1968.
49. Desmond, M. M., et al.: Congenital rubella encephalitis: Course and early sequelae. *J Pediatr, 71:*311, 1967.
50. Miller, J. W.: Timing of human congenital malformation. *Dev Med Child Neurol, 5:*343, 1963.
51. Macmahon, B. and Nazzan, L.: Ethnic difference in the presence of anencephaly and spina bifida in Boston, Massachusetts. *N Engl J Med, 277:*119, 1967.
52. Kilham, L. and Marzalis, G.: Pathogenicity of minute virus of mice (MVM) for rats, mice and hamsters. *Proc Soc Exp Biol Med, 133:*1447, 1970.
53. Johnson, R. T.: Effects of serial infections on the developing nervous system. *N Engl J Med, 287:*599, 1972.
54. Naege, R. I. and Blanc, W.: Pathogenesis of congenital rubella. *JAMA, 194:*1277, 1965.
55. Meyers, R. E.: Brain pathology following fetal vascular occlusion: An experimental study. *Invest Ophthal, 8:*41, 1969.
56. Crome, L.: Multilocular cystic encephalopathy of infants. *J Neurol Neurosurg Psychiat, 21:*146, 1958.
57. Kramer, W.: Multilocular encephalomalacia. *J Neurol Neurosurg Psychiat, 19:*209, 1956.
58. Overall, J. C., Jr., and Glasgreen, I. A.: Virus infections of the fetus and neurologic impact. *J Pediatr, 77:*315, 1970.
59. Berg, J. M. and Kuman, B. H.: Syphilis as a cause of neonatal deformity. *Br Med J, 2:*400, 1959.
60. Rugh, R.: Ionizing radiation and congenital anomalies of the nervous system. *Milit Med, 127:*883, 1962.
61. Miller, R. W.: Delayed radiation effects in atomic bomb survivors. *Science, 166:*369, 1969.

62. Hicks, S. P.: Developmental malformations produced by radiation. *Am J Roentgenol, 62:*272, 1953.
63. Dekalon, A. S.: Abnormalities in children exposed to x-radiation during various stages of gestation. Tentative timetable of radiation injury to the human fetus, Part I. *J Neurol Med, 9:*471, 1968.
64. Wood, J. W., Johnson, K. G. and Omori, Y.: In utero exposure to the Hiroshima atomic bomb: An evaluation of head size and mental retardation twenty years later. *Pediatrics, 39:*385, 1967.
65. Navarreti, V. N., et al.: Subsequent diabetes in mothers delivered of a malformed infant. *Lancet, 2:*993, 1976.
66. Eayes, J. T.: Endocrine influence on cerebral development. *Arch Biol, 75:*529, 1964.
67. LaFranchi, S. H., et al.: Neonatal hypothyroidism detected by northwest regional screening program. *Pediatrics, 63:*180, 1979.
68. Segal, S. et al.: Treatment of congenital hypothyroidism. *Pediatrics, 62:*413, 1978.
69. Rosman, N. P., Malone, A. J., Helfenstein, M., and Kroft, E.: The effect of thyroid deficiency on myelination of brain. *Neurology, 22:*99, 1972.
70. Ford, D. H.: Central nervous system — thyroid relationships. *Brain Res, 7:*329, 1968.
71. Rush, D., Stein, Z., and Susser, M.: A randomized control trial of prenatal nutritional supplementation in New York City. *Pediatrics, 65:*683, 1980.
72. Smith, D. W.: Recognizing patterns of human malformation. In Schaffer, A. J. (Ed.): *Major Problems in Clinical Pediatrics*, Philadelphia, Saunders, 1970, vol. VII.
73. Milunsky, A.: *The Prevention of Genetic Disease and Mental Retardation.* Philadelphia, Saunders, 1975.
74. Penrose, L. S.: Mongolism. *Br Med Bull, 17:*184, 1961.
75. Hsia, Y. E., Bratic, M., and Herboult, A.: Genetics of the Meckel syndrome. *Pediatrics, 48:*237, 1971.
76. Freeman, M. V. R., et al.: The Roberts syndrome. *Clin Genet, 5:*1, 1974.
77. Holmes, L. B., Driscoll, S. G., and Atkins, L.: Etiologic heterogeneity of neural tube defects. *N Engl J Med, 294:*365, 1976.
78. Allan, L. D., et al.: Amniotic fluid alpha-fetoprotein in the antenatal diagnosis of spina bifida. *Lancet, 2:*522, 1973.
79. Hamburger, V. and Habel, K.: Teratogenic and lethal effects of influenza-A and mumps viruses on early chick embryos. *Proc Soc Exp Biol Med, 66:*608, 1947.
80. Johnson, K. P., Klasnja, R., and Johnson, R. T.: Neural tube defects of chick embryos: An indirect result of influenza A virus infection. *J neuropathol Exp Neurol, 30:*68, 1971.
81. Robertson, G. G., Williamson, A. P., and Blatiner, R. J.: Origin of myeloschisis in chick embryos infected with influenza-A virus. *Yale J Biol Med, 32:*449, 1960.

82. Dekaban, A. S.: Anencephaly in early human embryos. *J Neuropathol Exp Neurol, 22:*533, 1963.

83. Beach, B.: Arnold-Chiari malformation. Anatomic features of 20 cases. *Arch Neurol, 12:*613, 1965.

84. Stagno, S., et al.: Auditory and visual defects resulting from symptomatic and subclinical congenital cytomegaloviral and *Toxoplasma* infections. *Pediatrics, 59:*669, 1977.

85. Dekaban, A. S.: Arhinencephaly. *Am J Ment Defic, 63:*428, 1948.

86. Schneck, L., Walk, B. W., and Saifer, A.: The gangliosidoses. *Am J Med, 46:*245, 1969.

87. Bodis-Wallner, I., Hendley, C. D., Mylin, L. H., and Thornton, J.: Visual evoked potentials and the visuogram in multiple sclerosis. *Ann Neurol, 5:*40, 1979.

88. Jacobson, M.: *Developmental Neurobiology.* New York, Holt, Rinehart, & Winston, 1970.

89. Adams, R. D. and Sedman, R. L.: *Introduction to Neuropathology.* New York, McGraw-Hill, 1968.

90. Osburn, B. I., et al.: Experimental viral-induced congenital encephalopathies I. Pathology of hydranencephaly and porencephaly caused by bluetongue vaccine virus. *Lab Invest, 25:*197, 1971.

91. Osburn, B. I., et al.: Experimental viral-induced congenital encephalopathies II. The pathogenesis of bluetongue vaccine virus infection in fetal lambs. *Lab Invest, 25:*206, 1971.

92. Kilham, L. and Margolin, G.: Cerebellar disease in cats induced by inoculation of rat virus. *Science, 148:*244, 1956.

93. Kilham, L. and Margolin, G.: Viral etiology of spontaneous ataxia of cats. *Am J Pathol, 48:*991, 1966.

94. Johnson, R. T., Johnson, K. P., and Edwards, C. J.: Virus induced hydrocephalus: Development of aqueductal stenosis in hamsters after mumps virus infection. *Science, 157:*1066, 1967.

95. Johnson, K. P. and Johnson, R. T.: Granular ependymitis: Occurrence in myxovirus infected rodents and prevalence in man. *Am J Pathol, 67:*511, 1972.

96. Bickers, D. S. and Adams, R. D.: Hereditary stenosis of the aqueduct of Sylvius as a cause of congenital hydrocephalus. *Brain, 72:*245, 1949.

97. Courville, C. B.: *Birth and Brain Damage.* Pasadena, Courvills, 1971.

98. Towbin, A.: Central nervous system damage in the human fetus and newborn infant. *Am J Dis Child, 119:*529, 1970.

99. Overall, S. G.: Neonatal bacterial meningitis. *J Pediatr, 76:*499, 1970.

100. Krayenbuchl, H. A.: Abscess of the brain. *Clin Neurosurg, 14:*25, 1966.

101. Blackwood, W. and Corsellis, J. A. W. (Eds.): *Greenfield's Neuropathology.* Chicago, Year Book Medical Publishers, 1976.

102. Avey, J. B. and Anderson, D. W.: Pathology of the newborn. In Greenhill, J. P. (Ed.): *Obstetrics.* Philadelphia, Saunders, 1965, pp. 247-311.

103. Mealey, J. Jr.: *Pediatric Head Injuries.* Springfield, Thomas, 1968.
104. Mealey, J. Jr.: Infantile subdural hematomas. *Ped Clin North Am, 22:*433, 1975.
105. Prensky, A. L., Dodge, P. R., Barlow, C., French, J. H., and Johnson, S. D.: Interrelationships between the nervous system and nutritional, electrolyte and endocrine disorders. In Swaiman, K. F. and Wright, F. S. (Eds.): *The Practice of Pediatric Neurology.* St. Louis, Mosby, 1975.
106. Towbin, A.: Cerebral hypoxic damage in fetus and newborn. *Arch Neurol, 20:*35, 1969.
107. Masland, R. L. In James, L. S., Myers, R. E., and Gaull, G. E. (Eds): Brain Damage in the Fetus and Newborn from Hypoxia or Asphyxia. Report of the Fifty-Seventh Ross Conference on Pediatric Research. Columbus, Ross Laboratories, 1967, pp. 110-112.
108. Smith, D. W., Blizard, R. M., and Wilkins, L.: The mental prognosis in hypothyroidism in infancy and childhood. *Pediatrics, 19:*1011, 1957.
109. Lloyd-Still, J. D., Hurwitz, I., Wolff, P. H., and Shrachman, H.: Intellectual development after severe malnutrition in infancy. *Pediatrics, 54:* 306, 1974.
110. American Academy for Cerebral Palsy: *Kernicterus and its Importance in Cerebral Palsy.* Springfield, Thomas, 1961.
111. Gartner, L. M., et al.: Kernicterus: High incidence in premature infants with low serum bilirubin concentration. *Pediatrics, 45:*906, 1970.
112. Sokoloff, L.: Circulation and energy metabolism of the brain. In Alhers, R. W., Siegel, G. J., Katzman, R. and Agrunoff, B. W.: *Basic Neurochemistry.* Boston, Little Brown, 1972, pp. 299-326.
113. Stanley, F. J. and Alberman, E. D.: Infants of very low birth weight. II Perinatal factors in and conditions associated with respiratory distress syndrome. *Dev Med Child Neurol, 20:*313, 1978.
114. Low, H. C., Shov, H., and Pedersen, H.: Low cerebral blood flow: A risk factor in the neonate. *J Pediatr, 95:*606, 1979.
115. Cooke, R. W. I., Rolfe, P., and Hovat, P.: Apparent cerebral blood flow in newborns with respiratory distress. *Dev Med Child Neurol, 21:*154, 1979.
116. Barmada, M. A., Morassy, J., and Shuman, R. M.: Cerebral infarcts with arterial occlusion in neonate. *Ann Neurol, 6:*495, 1979.
117. Banker, B. Q.: Cerebral vascular disease in infancy and childhood: I. Occlusive vascular disease. *J Neuropathol Exp Neurol, 20:*127, 1961.
118. Padger, D. H.: The development of the cranial arteries in the human embryo. *Carnegie Institution of Washington Contributions to Embryology, 32:*205, 1948.
119. Schadé, J. P. and McMenerney, W. M.: *Selective Vulnerability of the Brain in Hypoxemia.* Oxford, Blackwell Scientific, 1963.
120. Smith, A. and Sugar, O.: Development of above normal language and intelligence 21 years after left hemispherectomy. *Neurol, 25:*813, 1975.

121. Schadé, J. P. Muter, K., and Van Graeninjen, W. B.: Maturational aspects of the dendrites in the human cortex. *Acta Morph Neurol Scand*, 5:37, 1962.

122. Purpura, D. P.: Dendritic spine "dysgenesis" and mental retardation. *Science, 186:*1126, 1974.

123. Brachman, D. S., Hodges, F. J., and Freeman, J. M.: Computerized axial tomography in neurologic disorders of children. *Pediatrics, 59:*352, 1977.

124. Jasper, H. H., Ward, A. A. Jr., and Pope, A.: *Basic Mechanisms of the Epilepses.* Boston, Little Brown, 1969.

125. Huttenlocher, P. R.: Dendritic development in neocortex of children with mental defects and infantile spasms. *Neurol (Minneap.), 24:*203, 1974.

126. Purpura, D. P. and Suzuki, K.: Distortion of neuronal geometry and formation of aberrant synapses in neuronal storage disease. *Brain Res, 116:*1, 1976.

127. Gilles, F. H. and Murphy, S. F.: Perinatal telencephalic leucoencephalopathy. *J Neurol Neurosurg Psychiat, 32:*404, 1969.

128. Pansky, A. L., Carr, S., and Moser, H. W.: Development of myelin in inherited disorders of amino acid metabolism. *Arch Neurol, 19:*552, 1968.

129. Norton, W. T. and Poduslo, S. E.: Metachromatic leucodystrophy: Chemically abnormal myelin and cerebral biopsy studies of three siblings. In Ansell, G. B. (Ed.): *Variations in the Chemical Composition of the Nervous System.* Oxford, Pergamon, 1965, p. 82.

130. Hoffman, J. and Liss, H.: Hydranencephaly. *Acta Paedriatr Scand, 58:*297, 1969.

131. Naeye, R. L.: The epidemiology of perinatal mortality. The power of the autopsy. *Pediatr Clin North Am, 19:*295, 1972.

132. Harche, H. T., Jr., Naeye, R. L., Storch, A., and Blanc, W. A.: Perinatal cerebral intraventricular hemorrhage. *J Pediatr, 80:*37, 1972.

133. Towbin, A.: Central nervous system damage in the human fetus and newborn infant. *Am J Dis Child, 119:*529, 1970.

134. Towbin, A.: Cerebral intraventricular hemorrhage and subependymal matrix infarction in the fetus and premature newborn. *Am J Pathol, 52:*121, 1968.

135. MacGregor, A. R.: *Pathology of Infancy and Childhood.* Edinburgh, Livingston, 1960.

136. Fredrick, J. and Butler, N. R.: Certain causes of neonatal death II. Intraventricular hemorrhage. *Biol Neonate, 15:*257, 1970.

137. Larroche, J. C.: Post-haemorrhagic hydrocephalus in infancy: Anatomical study. *Biol Neonate, 20:*287, 1972.

138. Cutler, R. W. P., et al.: Formation and absorption of cerebrospinal fluid in man. *Brain, 91:*707, 1968.

139. Voris, H. C.: Postmeningitic hydrocephalus. *Neurology (Minneap.), 5:*72, 1955.

140. Russell, D. S.: Observations on the pathology of hydrocephalus. *Med Res Coune Spec Rep (London), 265:*1, 1949.

141. Goldstein, G. W., et al.: Transient hydrocephalus in premature infants, treatment by lumbar puncture. *Lancet, 1:*512, 1972.

142. Tsiantos, A., et al.: Intracranial hemorrhage in the prematurely born infant. *J. Pediatr, 85:*854, 1974.

143. Krishnamoorthy, K. S., et al.: Neurologic sequelae in the survivors of neonatal intraventricular hemorrhage. *Pediatrics, 64:*233, 1979.

144. Volpe, J.: Neonatal seizures. *N Engl J Med, 289:*413, 1973.

145. Tibbles, J. A. R. and Prichard, J. S.: The prognostic value of the electroencephalogram in neonatal convulsions. *Pediatrics, 35:*778, 1965.

146. Rose, A. L. and Lombroso, C. T.: Neonatal seizure states. *Pediatrics, 45:*404, 1970.

147. Lombrosco, C. T.: Seizures in the newborn period. In Vinkin, P. J. and Gruyn, G. W. (Eds.): *Handbook of Clinical Neurology.* New York, American Elsevier, 1974, vol. XV, pp. 187-218.

148. Burke, J. B.: The prognostic significance of neonatal convulsions. *Arch Dis Child, 29:*342, 1954.

149. Craig, W. S.: Convulsive movements occurring in the first ten days of life. *Arch Dis Child, 35:*336, 1960.

150. Freeman, J. M.: Neonatal seizures. In Swainman, K. F. and Wright, F. S. (Eds.): *The Practice of Pediatric Neurology.* St. Louis, Mosby, 1975, pp. 862-870.

151. Plum, F., Howe, D. C., and Duffy, T. E.: Metabolic effects of seizures. *Res Publ Assoc Res Nerv Ment Dis, 53:*141, 1974.

152. Wasterlain, C. G. and Plum, F.: Vulnerability of developing rat brain to electroconvulsive seizures. *Arch Neurol, 29:*38, 1973.

153. Wasterlain, C. G.: Effects of neonatal status epilepticus on rat brain development. *Neurology, 26:*975, 1976.

154. Bray, P., et al.: Occipitofrontal head circumference: An accurate measure of intracranial volume. *J Pediatr, 75:*303, 1969.

155. Buda, F. B., Reed, J. C., and Rabe, E. F.: Skull volume in infants: Methodology, normal values and application. *Am J Dis Child, 129:*1171, 1975.

156. Lubchenco, L. O., Hansman, M., and Boyd, E.: Intra-uterine growth in length and head circumference as estimated from live births at gestational ages from 26 to 42 weeks. *Pediatrics, 37:*403, 1966.

157. Sher, P. K. and Brown, S. B.: A longitudinal study of head growth in preterm infants I: Normal rates of head growth. *Dev Med Child Neurol, 17:*705, 1975.

158. Marks, K. H., et al.: Head growth in sick premature infants: A longitudinal study. *J Pediatr, 94:*282, 1979.

159. McCullough, D. C., Krofts, C., Axellman, S. P., and Schellinger, D.: Computerized axial tomography in clinical pediatrics. *Pediatrics, 59:*173, 1977.

160. Holmes, L. B., et al.: *Mental Retardation, An Atlas of Diseases with Associated Physical Abnormalities.* New York, Macmillan, 1972.

161. Gellis, S. S. and Feingold, M.: *Atlas of Mental Retardation Syndromes.* Washington, D.C., Department of Health, Education and Welfare, Rehabilitative Sciences Administration, Division of Mental Retardation, 1968.

162. Asch, A. J. and Myers, G. J.: Benign familial macrocephaly: Report of a family and review of the literature. *Pediatrics, 57:*535, 1976.

163. Danson, H.: Dynamic aspects of cerebrospinal fluid. *Dev Med Child Neurol, 14 (Suppl G):*1, 1972.

164. Dandy, W. E.: Diagnosis and treatment of strictures of the aqueduct of Sylvius (causing hydrocephalus). *Arch Surg (Chicago), 51:*1, 1945.

165. Dandy, W. E.: Diagnosis and treatment of hydrocephalus due to occlusion of the foramina of Magendie and Luschka. *Surg Gynecol Obstet, 32:*112, 1921.

166. Peach, B.: Arnold-Chiari malformation: Morphogenesis. *Arch Neurol, 12:*527, 1965.

167. Cameron, A. H.: Arnold-Chiari and other neuroanatomical malformations associated with spina bifida. *J Pathol Bacteriol, 73:*195, 1957.

168. Russell, D. S. and Donald, G.: The mechanism of internal hydrocephalus in spina bifida. *Brain, 58:*203, 1935.

169. Padget, D. H.: Development of so-called dystrophism with embryologic evidence of clinical Arnold-Chiari and Dandy-Walker malformations. *Johns Hopkins Med J, 130:*127, 1972.

170. Nixon, G. W., Johns, R. E., Jr., and Myers, G. G.: Congenital porencephaly. *Pediatrics, 54:*43, 1974.

171. Chamberlain, W. E.: Basilar impression (platybasia) a bizarre developmental anomaly of the occipital bone and upper cervical spine with striking and misleading neurologic manifestation. *Yale J Biol Med, 11:*489, 1939.

172. Gunderson, C. H., Greenspan, R. H., Glaser, G. H., and Lubs, H. A.: The Klippel-Feil syndrome: Genetic and clinical re-evaluation of cervical fusion. *Medicine, 46:*491, 1967.

173. Green, W. T.: The surgical correction of congenital elevation of the scapula (Sprengel's deformity). *J Bone Joint Surg, 37:A:*1439, 1957.

174. Matson, D. D.: *Neurosurgery of Infancy and Childhood,* 2nd ed. Springfield, Thomas, 1969.

175. Laurence, K. M., Hoarc, R. D., and Tell, K.: Diagnosis of the choroid plexus papilloma of the lateral ventricle. *Brain, 84:*628, 1961.

176. Hanshaw, J. B.: Congenital and acquired cytomegalic infection. *Pediatr Clin North Am, 13:*279, 166.

177. Pochedly, C.: Neurologic manifestations in acute leukemia. I Symptoms due to increased cerebrospinal fluid pressure and hemorrhage. *NY State J Med, 14:*575, 1975.

178. Hooper, R.: Hydrocephalus and obstruction of the superior vena cava in infancy. *Pediatrics, 28:*792, 1961.

179. Russell, D. S. and Beck, D. J. K.: Experiments on thrombosis of the superior longitudinal sinus. *J Neurosurg, 3:*337, 1946.

180. Schlessinger, B.: The tolerance of the blocked galenic system against artificially increased intracranial pressure. *Brain, 63:*178, 1940.

181. Rabe, E. F., Flynn, R. E., and Dodge, P. R.: Subdural collections of fluid in infants and children. *Neurology (Minneap.), 18:*559, 1968.

182. Follis, R. H.: Osteogenesis imperfecta congenita: A connective tissue diasthesis. *J Pediatr, 41:*713, 1952.

183. Smith, C. H.: *Blood Diseases of Infancy and Childhood,* 3rd ed. St. Louis, Mosby, 1972.

184. Behrman, R. E. (Ed.): *Neonatology.* St. Louis, Mosby, 1973.

185. Dennis, J. P., Rosenberg, H. A., and Alvard, E. G., Jr.: Megalencephaly, internal hydrocephalus and other neurological aspects of achondroplasia. *Brain, 84:*427, 1961.

186. Sotos, J. F., et al.: Cerebral gigantism in childhood. *N Engl J Med, 271:*109, 1964.

187. Grant, D. N.: Benign intracranial hypertension. *Arch Dis Child, 46:*651, 1971.

188. Wilson, S. A. K.: Megalencephaly. *J Neurol Psychopathol, 14:*193, 1934.

189. Benda, C. E.: *Developmental Disorders of Mentation and Cerebral Palsies.* New York, Grune & Stratton, 1952.

190. Bork, J. A., Schert, J. W., and Reed, A. C.: A clinical and genetical study of microcephaly. *Am J Ment Defic, 57:*637, 1953.

191. Connolly, C. J.: The fissural pattern of the primitive brain. *Am J Phys Anthrop, 21:*301, 1936.

192. Druckman, R., Chao, D., and Alvord, E. C., Jr.: A case of atonic cerebral diplegia with lissencephaly. *Neurology (Minneap.), 9:*806, 1959.

193. Cockayne, E. A.: Dwarfism with retinal atrophy and deafness. *Arch Dis Child, 11:*1, 1930.

194. Macdonald, W. B., Fitch, K. D., and Lewis, I. C.: Cockayne's syndrome. *Pediatrics, 25:*997, 1960.

195. Lawrence, K. M. and Cavanagh, J. B.: Progressive degeneration of the cortex in infancy. *Brain, 91:*261, 1968.

196. Haslam, R. H. S. and Smith, D. W.: Autosomal dominant microcephaly. *J Pediatr 95:*701, 1979.

197. Menkes, et al.: A sex-linked recessive disorder with retardation of growth, peculiar hair and focal cerebellar degeneration. *Pediatrics, 29:*764, 1962.

198. Streissguth, A. P., Herman, C. S., and Smith, D. W.: Intelligence, behavior and dysmorphogenesis in the fetal alcohol syndrome: A report on 20 patients. *J Pediatr, 92:*363, 1978.

199. Berman, P. H. and Banker, B. Q.: Neonatal meningitis: A clinical and pathological study of 29 cases. *Pediatrics, 38:*6, 1966.

200. Light, I. J.: Postnatal acquisition of Herpes simplex virus by the newborn infant: A review of the literature. *Pediatrics, 63:*480, 1979.

201. Anderson, H. and Gomes, S. P.: Craniosynostosis. *Acta Paediatr Scand, 57:*47, 1968.

202. Freeman, J. M. and Berkauf, S.: Craniosynostosis: Review of the literature and report of thirty-four cases. *Pediatrics, 30:*57, 1962.

203. Tempkin, O.: *The Falling Sickness.* Baltimore, Johns Hopkins, 1945.

204. Jasper, H. H., Ward, A. A., and Pope, A.: *Basic Mechanism of the Epilepsies.* Boston, Little Brown, 1969.

205. Cobb, S.: Causes of epilepsy. *Arch Neurol Psychiatr, 27:*1245, 1932.

206. Dodge, P. R.: Febrile convulsions. *J Pediatr, 78:*1083, 1971.

207. Millichap, S. G.: *Febrile Convulsions.* New York, Macmillan, 1968.

208. Patrick, H. T. and Lenz, D. M.: Early convulsions in epileptics and others. *JAMA, 82:*375, 1924.

209. Tower, D. B.: *Neurochemistry of Epilepsy Seizure Mechanisms and Their Management.* Springfield, Thomas, 1960.

210. Vandenberg, B. J. and Yerushaling, J.: Studies on convulsive disorders in young children (Incidence of febrile and nonfebrile convulsions by age and other factors). *Pediatr Rev, 3:*298, 1969.

211. Nelson, K. B. and Ellenberg, J. H.: Prognosis in children with febrile seizures. *Pediatrics, 61:*720, 1978.

212. Thorn, I.: A controlled study of prophylactic long term treatment of febrile convulsions with phenobarbital. *Acta Neurol Scand, 60 (Suppl):*67, 1975.

213. Kooi, K. A.: *Fundamentals of Electroencephalography.* New York, Harper & Row, 1971.

214. Lazy, S.: Assessment of a clinical and electroencephalographic classification of epileptic patients in everyday neurological practice: A survey of 450 cases. *Epilepsia, 13:*458, 1972.

215. Millichap, J. G.: Electroencephalography and other diagnostic procedures in epilepsy. *Modern Treat, 6:*1177, 1969.

216. Roger, J., Lab, H., and Tassenari, H.: Status epilepticus. In Vinkin, P. J. and Bruyn, G. W. (Eds.): *Handbook of Clinical Neurology.* New York, American Elsevier, 1974, vol. XV, pp. 145-188.

217. Millichap, J. G.: Drug treatment of convulsive disorders. *N Engl J Med, 286:*464, 1972.

218. Lombroso, C. T.: The treatment of status epilepticus. *Pediatrics, 53:*536, 1974.

219. Toman, J. E. P.: Drugs effective in convulsive disorders. In Goodman, L. S. and Gilman, A. (Eds.): *The Pharmacological Basis of Therapeutics,* 4th ed. London, Macmillan, 1970, pp. 204-225.

220. Arcardi, J. and Chevrie, J. J.: Convulsive status epilepticus in infants and children: A study of 239 cases. *Epilepsia, 11:*187, 1970.

221. Vajda, F. J. E., et al.: Rectal administration of sodium valproate in status epilepticus. *Neurology, 28:*897, 1978.
222. Singer, W. D., Rabe, E. F., and Haller, J. S.: The effect of ACTH therapy upon infantile spasms. *J Pediatr, 96:*485, 1980.
223. Gastaut, H., et al.: Childhood epileptic encephalopathy with diffuse slow spike-waves (otherwise known as "petit mal variant") or Lennox syndrome. *Epilepsia, 7:*139, 1966.
224. Markand, O. N.: Slow spike-wave activity in EEG and associated clinical features: Often called "Lennox" or "Lennox-Gastaut" syndrome. *Neurology (Minneap.), 27:*746, 1977.
225. Hanson, R. A. and Menkes, J. H.: A new anticonvulsant in the management of minor motor seizures. *Dev Med Child Neurol, 14:*3, 1972.
226. Hooshong, H.: Intractable seizures. *Arch Neurol, 27:*205, 1972.
227. Goldenberg, M. A. and Dorman, J. D.: Intention myoclonus — successful treatment with clonazepam. *Neurol, 26:*24, 1976.
228. Lance, J. W. and Anthony, M.: Clonazepam and sodium valproate in the treatment of intractable epilepsy. *Arch Neurol, 34:*14, 1977.
229. Adams, D. J., Luders, H. and Pippenger, C.: Sodium valproate in the treatment of intractable seizure disorders. *Neurol, 28:*152, 1978.
230. Mattson, R. H., Cramer, J. A., Williamson, P. D., and Novelly, R. A.: Valproic acid in epilepsy: Clinical and pharmacological effects. *Ann Neurol, 3:*20, 1978.
231. Browne, T. R.: Valproic acid. *N Engl J Med, 302:*661, 1980.
232. Batalden, P. B., VanDyne, B. J. and Cloyd, J.: Pancreatitis associated with valproic acid therapy. *Pediatrics, 64:*520, 1979.
233. Hyman, N. M., Dennis, P. D., and Sinclair, K. G. A.: Tremor due to sodium valproate. *Neurology (Minneap.), 29:*1177, 1979.
234. Dodson, W. E., et al.: Management of seizure disorders: Selected aspects part I. *J Pediatr, 89:*527, 1976.
235. Mattson, R. H., Cramer, J. A., Williamson, P. D. and Moselly, R. A.: Valproic acid in epilepsy: Clinical and pharmacological effects. *Ann Neurol, 3:*20, 1978.
236. Halowach, J., Thurston, D. L. and O'Leary, J.: Prognosis in childhood epilepsy: Follow-up study of 148 cases in which therapy has been suspended after prolonged anticonvulsant control. *N Engl J Med, 286:*169, 1972.
237. Rabe, E. F.: Anticonvulsant therapy: To stop or not to stop. *N Engl J Med, 286:*213, 1972.
238. Borgstedt, A. D., Bryson, M. F., Young, L. W., and Forbes, G. B.: Long term administration of antiepileptic drugs and the development of rickets. *J Pediatr, 81:*9, 1972.
239. Medlensky, H. L.: Rickets associated with anticonvulsant medication. *Pediatrics, 53:*91, 1974.
240. Matsuda, I., et al.: Renal tubular acidosis and skeletal demineralization in patients on long term anticonvulsant therapy. *J Pediatr, 87:*202, 1975.

241. Tolman, K. G., et al.: Osteomalacia associated with anticonvulsant drug therapy in mentally retarded children. *Pediatrics, 56:*45, 1975.

242. Crosby, C. J., Chee, C., and Berman, P. H.: Rickets associated with long term anticonvulsant therapy in a pediatric outpatient population. *Pediatrics, 56:*52, 1975.

243. Benda, C. E.: *Developmental Disorders of Mentation and Cerebral Palsy.* New York, Grune & Stratton, 1952.

244. Swinyard, C. H., Swensen, L., and Greenspan, L.: An institutional survey of 143 cases of acquired cerebral palsy. *Dev Med Child Neurol, 5:*615, 1963.

245. Ingram, T. T. S.: *Paediatric Aspects of Cerebral Palsy.* Edinburgh, Tennystone, 1964.

246. Crothers, B. and Paine, R. S.: *The Natural History of Cerebral Palsy.* Cambridge, Harvard University Press, 1959.

247. Hansen, E.: Cerebral palsy in Denmark. *Acta Psychiatr Scand, 35 (Suppl 146):*1, 1960.

248. Minear, W. L. A.: A classification of cerebral palsy. *Pediatrics, 18:*841, 1956.

249. Ford, F. R.: *Diseases of the Nervous System in Infancy Childhood and Adolescence,* 6th ed. Springfield, Thomas, 1973.

250. Worster-Draught, C.: Congenital suprabulbar paresis. *J Laryngol, 70:*453, 1956.

251. Freytag, E. and Lindenberg, R.: Neuropathological findings in patients of a hospital for the mentally deficient: A survey of 359 cases. *Johns Hopkins Med J, 121:*3791, 1967.

252. Malamud, N., et al.: An etiologic and diagnostic study of cerebral palsy. *J Pediatr, 65:*270, 1964.

253. Marin-Padilla, M.: Structural abnormalities of the cerebral cortex in human chromosome aberrations. A Golgi study. *Brain Res, 44:*625, 1972.

254. Tobin, A.: *The Pathology of Cerebral Palsy.* Springfield, Thomas, 1960.

255. Peterson, H. A. and Coventry, M. B.: Long-term results of surgical treatment of adults with cerebral palsy. *Dev Med Child Neurol, 11:*35, 1969.

256. Wright, T. and Nicholson, J.: Physiotherapy for the spastic child: An evaluation. *Dev Med Child Neurol, 15:*146, 1973.

257. Piper, M. C. and Pless, I. B.: Early intervention for infants with Down syndrome: A controlled trial. *Pediatrics, 65:*463, 1980.

258. Cruickshank, W. M. (Ed.): *Cerebral Palsy, A Developmental Disability.* Syracuse, University Press, 1976.

259. Twitchell, T. E.: Variations and abnormalities of motor development. *J Am Phy Therap Assoc, 45:*424, 1963.

260. Twitchell, T. E.: On the motor deficits in congenital bilateral athetosis. *J Nerv Ment Dis, 129:*105, 1959.

261. Twitchell, T. E.: The grasping deficit in infantile spastic hemiparesis. *Neurol (Minneap.), 8:*13, 1958.

262. Twitchell, T. E.: The nature of the motor deficit in double athetosis. *Arch Phys Med Rehab, 42:*63, 1961.

263. Rabe, E. F.: The hypotonic infant: A review. *J Pediatr, 64:*422, 1964.

264. Swaiman, K. F. and Wright, F. S.: *Neuromuscular Diseases in Infancy and Childhood.* Springfield, Thomas, 1970.

265. Eldred, E. and Buchwald, J.: Central nervous system: Motor mechanisms. *Ann Rev Physiol, 29:*573, 1967.

266. Wright, F. S.: An approach to hypotonia in children. *Postgrad Med, 50:*116, 1971.

267. Pearce, J. M. S., Pennington, R. T., and Walton, J. N.: Serum enzyme studies in muscle disease: Part II Serum creatine kinase activity in muscular dystrophy and neuropathic disorders. *J Neurol Neurosurg Psychiat, 27:*96, 1964.

268. Lambert, E. H.: Neurophysiological techniques useful in the study of neuromuscular disorders. *Res Proc Assoc Nerv Ment Dis, 38:*247, 1958.

269. Bethlem, J.: *Muscle Pathology.* Amsterdam, North Holland, 1970.

270. Van Praugh: Diagnosis of kernicterus in the neonatal period. *Pediatrics, 28:*870, 1961.

271. Wright, F. S.: Hypotonia. In Swaiman, K. F. and Wright, F. S.: *The Practice of Pediatric Neurology.* St. Louis, Mosby, 1975, pp. 214-217.

272. Gamstorp, I.: Progressive spinal muscular atrophy without onset in infancy or early childhood. *Acta Paediatr Scand, 56:*408, 1967.

273. Byers, R. K. and Banker, B. Q.: Infantile muscular atrophy. *AMA Arch Neurol, 5:*140, 1961.

274. Kugelberg, E. and Welander, L.: Hereditofamilial juvenile muscular atrophy simulating muscular dystrophy. *Arch Neurol Psychiat, 75:*500, 1956.

275. Tsukagorki, H., et al.: Kugelberg-Welander syndrome with dominant inheritance. *Arch Neurol, 14:*378, 1966.

276. Bodian, D. and Horstimann, D. M.: Polioviruses. In Horsfall, F. L. and Tamm, I. (Eds.): *Viral and Rickettsial Infections of Man.* Philadelphia, Lippincott, 1965.

277. Melneck, J. L., Wenner, H. A., and Posen, L.: Enteroviruses. In Lennette, E. H. and Schmidt, N. J. (Eds.): *Diagnostic Procedures for Viral and Rickettsial Infections,* 4th ed. New York, American Public Health Association, 1969.

278. Drachman, D. B. and Banker, B. Q.: Arthrogryposis multiplex congenita. *AMA Arch Neurol, 5:*89, 1961.

279. Williams, P. F.: The early correction of deformities in arthrogryposis multiplex congenita. *Aust Ped J, 2:*194, 1966.

280. McFarland, H. R. and Heller, G. L.: Guillain-Barre disease complex. *Arch Neurol, 14:*196, 1966.

281. Eberle, E., Brink, J., Azen, S. and White, D.: Early prediction of incomplete recovery in children with Guillain-Barre polyneuritis. *J Pediatr, 86:*356, 1975.

282. Byers, R. K. and Taft, L. T.: Chronic multiple peripheral neuropathy in childhood. *Pediatrics, 40:*517, 1957.

283. Gilroy, J. and Meyers, J. S.: *Medical Neurology.* London, Macmillan, 1969, pp. 183-191.

284. Osserman, K. E.: *Myasthenia Gravis.* New York, Grune & Stratton, 1958.

285. Strickroot, F. I., Schaeffer, R. L. and Berger, H. L.: Myasthenia gravis occurring in an infant born of a myasthenic mother. *JAMA, 120:*1207, 1942.

286. Millichap, J. G. and Dodge, P. R.: Diagnosis and treatment of myasthenia gravis in infancy, childhood and adolescence. *Neurology, 10:*1007, 1960.

287. Drachman, D. B.: Myasthenia gravis, Parts I & II. *N Engl J Med, 298:*130 & 186, 1978.

288. Eitzman, D. and Wolfson, S. E.: Acute parathion poisoning in children. *Am J Dis Child, 114:*397, 1967.

289. Koenig, M. G., et al.: Type B botulism in man. *Am J Med, 42:*208, 1967.

290. Pickett, J., Berg, B., Chaplin, E., Brunstetter, and Shafer, M.: Syndrome of botulism in infancy: Clinical and electrophysiologic study. *N Engl J Med, 295:*770, 1976.

291. Short, J. K.: Congenital muscular dystrophy: A case report with autopsy findings. *Neurology, 13:*526, 1963.

292. Turner, J. W. A. and Lees, F.: Congenital myopathy: A 50 year follow-up. *Brain, 85:*733, 1962.

293. Munsat, T. L. and Pearson, C. M.: The differential diagnosis of neuro-muscular weakness in infancy and childhood. Part II. The dystrophic myopathies. *Dev Med Child Neurol, 9:*319, 1967.

294. Dodge, P. R., Gamstorp, I., Byers, R. K., and Russell, P.: Myotonic dys-trophy in infancy and childhood. *Pediatrics, 35:*3, 1965.

295. Wedgeward, R. J. P., Cook, C., and Cohen, J.: Dematomyositis: Report of 26 cases in children with a discussion of endocrine therapy in 13. *Pediatrics, 12:*447, 1953.

296. Pearson, C. M.: Polymyositis. *Ann Rev Med, 17:*63, 1966.

297. Gould, S. E.: *Trichinosis.* Springfield, Thomas, 1945.

298. Shy, G. M., et al.: Nemaline myopathy: A new congenital myopathy. *Brain, 86:*793, 1963.

299. Shy, G. M. and Majeu, K. R.: A new congenital non-progressive myopathy. *Brain, 79:*610, 1956.

300. Spiro, A. J., Shy, G. M., and Gonatas, N. K.: Myotubular myopathy. *Arch Neurol, 14:*1, 1966.

301. Shy, G. M., Gavatas, N. K., and Perey, M.: Two childhood myopathies with abnormal mitochondria. *Brain, 89:*133, 1966.

302. MacDonald, R. D., Rewrastle, L. B., and Humphrey, J. G.: Myopathy of hypokalemic periodic paralysis. *Arch Neurol, 20:*565, 1969.

303. Brooks, J. E.: Hyperkalemic periodic paralysis. *Arch Neurol, 20:*13, 1969.

304. McArdle, B.: Myopathy due to a defect in muscle glycogen breakdown. *Clin Sci, 10:*13, 1951.

305. Layzer, R. B., Rowland, I. P., and Ranney, H. M.: Muscle phosphofructokinase deficiency. *Arch Neurol, 17:*512, 1967.

306. Rowland, I. P., et al.: Myoglobinuria. *Arch Neurol, 10:*537, 1964.

307. Walton, J. N.: The limp child. *J Neurol Neurosurg Psychiat, 20:*144, 1957.

308. Walton, J. N.: Amyotonia congenita, a follow-up study. *Lancet, 1:*1023, 1956.

309. Buda, F. B., Rothney, W. B., and Rabe, E. F.: Hypotonia and the maternal child relationship. *Am J Dis Child, 124:*906, 1972.

310. Kanner, L.: Autistic disturbances of affective content. *Nerv Child, 2:*217, 1943.

311. Rutter, M.: Concepts in autism: A review of research. *J Child Psychol Psychiat, 9:*1, 1968.

312. Knoblack, H. and Pasamoneck, B.: Some etiologic and prognostic factors in early infantile autism and psychoses. *Pediatrics, 55:*182, 1975.

313. Knoblack, H. and Kerr-Grant, D.: Etiologic factors in "early infantile autism" and "childhood schizophrenia" *Am J Dis Child, 102:*535, 1961.

314. Goldfarb, W.: *Childhood Schizophrenia.* Cambridge, Harvard University Press, 1961.

315. Ornitz, E. M. and Ritso, E. R.: Perceptual inconsistencies in infantile autism. *Arch Gen Psychiat, 18:*76, 1968.

316. Spitz, R. A.: The psychogenic disease in infancy. *Psychoanal Study Child, 6:*255, 1951.

317. Bender, L.: Childhood schizophrenia, clinical study of 100 schizophrenic children. *Am J Orthopsychiat, 17:*40, 1947.

318. Wing, J.: *Early Childhood Autism: Clinical Educational and School Aspects.* London, Pergamon Press, 1966.

319. Bettelheim, B.: *The Empty Fortress. Infantile Autism and the Birth of the Self.* London, Collier-Macmillian, 1967.

320. Lockyer, L. and Rutter, M.: A five to fifteen year follow-up study of infantile psychosis: III Psychological aspects. *Br J Psychiat, 115:*865, 1969.

321. Cunningham, M. A.: A five year study of the language of an autistic child. *J Child Psychol Psychiat, 7:*143, 1966.

322. Eisenberg, L. and Kanner, L.: Early infantile autism 1943-55. *Am J Orthopsychiat, 26:*556, 1956.

323. Rimland, B.: *Infantile Autism.* New York, Appleton-Century-Crofts, 1964.

324. Salamy, A., McKean, C. M., and Buda, F. B.: Maturational changes in auditory transmission as reflected in human brain stem potentials. *Brain Res, 96:*361, 1975.

325. Schain, R. J. and Yannet, H.: Infantile autism: An analysis of 50 cases and a consideration of certain neurophysiologic concepts. *J Pediatr, 57:*560, 1960.

326. White, P. T., DeMeyer, W., and DeMeyer, M.: EEG abnormalities in early childhood schizophrenia: A double blend study of psychiatrically disturbed and normal children during promazine sedation. *Am J Psychiat. 120:*950, 1964.

327. Tanguay, P. E.: A pediatrician's guide to the recognition and initial treatment of early infantile autism. *Pediatrics, 51:*903, 1973.

328. Swanson, J., Kinsbourne, M., Roberts, W., and Zurker, K.: Time response analysis of the effect of stimulant medication on the learning ability of children referred for hyperactivity. *Pediatrics, 61:*21, 1978.

329. Solomons, G.: Guidelines on the use and medical effects of psychostimulant drugs in therapy. *J Learn Dis, 4:*6, 1971.

330. Conners, C. K.: A teacher rating scale for use in drug studies with children. *Am J Psychiat, 126:*884, 1969.

331. Conners, C. K.: Psychological assessment of children with minimal brain dysfunction. *Ann N Y Acad Sci, 205:*283, 1973.

332. Davids, A.: An objective instrument for assessing hyperkinesis in children. *J Learn Dis, 4:*35, 1971.

333. Denhoff, E., Davids, A., and Hawkins, R.: Effects of dextroamphetamines on hyperkinetic children: A controlled double-blind study. *J Learn Dis, 4:*27, 1971.

334. Wolraich, M. L.: Stimulant drug therapy in hyperactive children: Research and clinical implementation. *Pediatrics, 60:*512, 1977.

335. Alexandris, A. and Lundell, F. W.: Effect of thioridazine, amphetamine and placebo on the hyperkinetic syndrome and cognitive area in mentally deficient children. *Can Med Assoc J, 98:*92, 1968.

336. Howell, M. C., et al.: Hyperactivity in children: Types, diagnosis drug therapy approaches to management. *Clin Pediatr, 11:*30, 1972.

337. Box, M.: The active and the overactive school child. *Dev Med Child Neurol, 14:*83, 1972.

338. Task Force on Nomenclature and Statistics: *Diagnostic and Statistical Manual of Mental Disorders,* 3rd ed (draft). Washington, American Psychiatric Association, 1978, pp. M26-M30.

339. Shaynitz, B. A., Cohen, D. J., and Shaynitz, S. E.: New diagnostic terminology for minimal brain dysfunction. *J Pediatr, 95:*734, 1979.

340. Charles, L., Schain, R. J., Zeiniker, T., and Guthrie, D.: Effects of methylphenerdate on hyperactive children's ability to sustain attention. *Pediatrics, 64:*412, 1979.

341. Shause, M. N. and Lubar, J. F.: Physiological basis of hyperkinesis treated with methylphenerdate. *Pediatrics, 62:*343, 1978.

342. Segundo, J. P., Aranz, R., and French, J. D.: Behavioral arousal by stimulation of the brain in the monkey. *J Neurosurg, 12:*601, 1955.

343. Conners, C. K.: Symposium: Behavior modification by drugs. II Psychological effects of stimulant drugs in children with minimal brain dysfunction. *Pediatrics, 49:*702, 1972.

344. Schain, R. J. and Reynard, C. L.: Effects of stimulant drugs (methyl-

phenerdate) in children with hyperactive behavior. *Pediatrics, 55:*709, 1975.

345. Eisenberg, L.: The clinical use of stimulant drugs in children. *Pediatrics, 49:*709, 1972.

346. Gross, M. D.: Growth of hyperkinetic children taking methylphenerdate, dextramphetamine or impramine/despramine. *Pediatrics, 58:*423, 1976.

347. Safer, D., Allen, R., and Barr, E.: Depression of growth in hyperactive children on stimulant drugs. *N Engl J Med, 287:*217, 1972.

348. Epstein, L. C., et al.: Correlation of dextroamphetamine excretion and drug response in hyperactive children. *J Nerv Ment Dis, 146:*136, 1968.

349. Laufer, M. W.: Long-term management and some follow-up findings on the use of drugs with minimal cerebral dysfunction. *J Learn Dis, 4:*518, 1971.

350. Safer, D. J., Allen, R. P., and Barr, E.: Growth rebound after termination of stimulant drugs. *J Pediatr, 86:*113, 1975.

351. Aarskoy, D., et al.: The effect of the stimulant drugs, dextraoamphetamine and methylphenidate on secretion of growth hormone in hyperactive children. *J Pediatr, 91:*136, 1977.

352. Dickinson, L. E.: Impaired growth in hyperactive children receiving pemoline. *J Pediatr, 94:*538, 1979.

353. Strauss, A. A. and Lehtinen, L. E.: *Psychopathology and Education of the Brain-Injured Child.* New York, Grune & Stratton, 1947.

354. Kahn, E. and Cohen, L. H.: Organic driveness: A brain stem syndrome and on experience. *N Engl J Med, 210:*748, 1934.

355. Clements, S. D. and Peters, J. E.: Minimal brain dysfunction in the school age child. *Arch Gen Psychiat, 6:*185, 1962.

356. Paine, R. S.: Minimal chronic brain syndrome in children. *Dev Med Child Neurol, 4:*21, 1962.

357. Lerer, R. J. and Lerer, M. P.: The effects of methylphenidate on the soft neurological signs of hyperactive children. *Pediatrics, 57:*521, 1976.

358. Schmitt, B. D., et al.: The hyperactive child. *Clin Pediatr, 12:*154, 1973.

359. Feingold, B., German, D. F., Braham, R. M., and Simmers, E.: Adverse reaction to food additive. Read before the annual convention of the American Medical Association, New York, 1973.

360. Williams, J. I., et al.: Relative effects of drugs and diet on hyperactive behavior: An experimental study. *Pediatrics, 61:*811, 1978.

361. Conners, C. K., et al.: Food additives and hyperkinesis: A controlled double blind experiment. *Pediatrics, 58:*154, 1976.

362. Shaywitz, S. E., Cohon, D. J., and Shaywitz, B. A.: The biochemical basis of minimal brain dysfunction. *J Pediatr, 92:*179, 1978.

363. Shetty, T. and Chase, T. N.: Central monoamines and hyperkinesis of childhood. *Neurology, 26:*1000, 1976.

364. Shaywitz, B. A., Goldenring, J. R., and Wool, R. S.: The effects of chron-

ic administration of food coloring on activity levels and cognitive performance in normal and hyperactive rat pups: Presented at Child Neurology Society Meeting, Dillon, Colorado, 1978.

365. Torgesen, J.: Problems and prospects in the study of learning disabilities. In Netherington, E. M. (Ed.): *Review of Child Development Research.* Chicago, University of Chicago Press, 1975, vol. V, pp. 385-440.

366. Kalvertoer, A. F.: *A Neurobehavioral Study in Pre-School Children, Clinics in Developmental Medicine,* No. 54. Philadelphia, Lippincott, 1975.

367. Tarnopal, L. and Tarnopal, M. (Eds.): *Brain Function and Reading Disabilities.* Baltimore, University Park Press, 1977.

368. LeDoux, J. E., Barclay, L., and Premack, A.: The brain and cognitive science. *Ann Neurol, 4:*391, 1978.

369. Sabatino, D. A. and Becker, J. T.: Relationship between lateral preference and selected behavioral variables for children failing academically. *Child Develop, 42:*2055, 1971.

370. Annett, M.: Handedness, cerebral dominance and the growth of intelligence. In Bakker, D. J. and Satz, P. (Eds.): *Specific Reading Disability.* Rotterdam, Rotterdam University Press, 1970.

371. Zangwill, O. L.: Dyslexia in relation to cerebral dominance. In Money, J. (Ed.): *Reading Disability: Progress and Research Needs in Dyslexia.* Baltimore, Johns Hopkins Press, 1962.

372. Kinsbourne, M.: Developmental Gerstmann syndrome: A disorder of sequencing. *Pediatr Clin North Am, 15:*771, 1968.

373. Birch, H. G. and Belmont, L.: Auditory-visual integration in retarded readers. *Am J Orthopsychiat, 34:*852, 1964.

374. Boder, E.: Developmental dyslexia: Prevailing diagnostic concepts and a new diagnostic approach through patterns of reading and spelling. In Myklebust, H. R. (Ed.): *Progress in Learning Disabilities.* New York, Grune & Stratton, 1971, vol. II.

375. Reed, E. W. and Reed, S. C.: *Mental Retardation, A Family Study.* Philadelphia, Saunders, 1965, pp. 1-82.

376. Dingman, H. F. and Taijan, G.: Mental retardation and the normal distribution curve. *Am J Ment Def, 64:*991, 1960.

377. Rutter, M.: Psychological development — predictors from infancy. In Chase, S. and Thomas, A. (Eds.): *Annual Progress in Child Psychiatry and Child Development.* New York, Brenner, Mazel, 1971.

378. Rosenfeld, G. B. and Bradley, C.: Childhood behavior sequelae of asphyxia in infancy. *Pediatrics, 2:*74, 1948.

379. Chess, S., Fernandez, P. and Korn, S.: Behavioral consequences of congenital rubella. *J Pediatr, 93:*699, 1978.

380. Fraser, M. S. and Wilks, J.: The residual effects of neonatal asphyxia. *J Obstet Gynecol Br Comm, 66:*748, 1959.

381. Levy, S.: Postencephalitis behavior disorder, a forgotten entity. *Am J Psychiat, 115:*1062, 1959.

382. Galahurde, A. M. and Kemper, T. L.: Cytoarchetectonic abnormalities in developmental dyslexia: A case study. *Ann Neurol, 6:*94, 1979.
383. Hier, D. B., et al.: Developmental dyslexia. *Arch Neurol, 35:*90, 1978.
384. Knoblack, H. and Pasamanich, B.: Syndrome of minimal cerebral damage in infancy. *JAMA, 170:*1384, 1959.
385. Wender, P. H.: *Minimal Brain Dysfunction in Children.* New York, Wiley, 1971.
386. Arnold, L. E. and Knopp: The making of a myth. *JAMA, 223:*1273, 1973.
387. Krager, J. M. and Safer, D. J.: Type and prevalence of medication used in the treatment of hyperactive children. *N Engl J Med, 291:*1118, 1974.
388. Pincus, J. H. and Glaser, G. H.: The syndrome of "minimal brain damage" in childhood. *N Engl J Med, 275:*27, 1966.
389. MacKeith, R. C. and Box, M.: *Minimal Cerebral Dysfunction.* Papers from the international study group held at Oxford, Sept 1962. London, Heinemann, 1963.
390. Gubbay, S. S., et al.: Clumsy children: A study of apraxic and agnostic defects in 21 children. *Brain, 88:*293, 1965.
391. Hecaen, H. and de Ajuriaguerr, J.: *Left-Handedness.* New York, Grune & Stratton, 1964.
392. Early identification of children with learning disabilities. Statement: American Academy of Pediatrics, November 1973.
393. Bayly, N.: Comparison of mental and motor test scores for age 1-15 months by sex, birth order, race, geographic location and education of parents. *Child Dev, 36:*378, 1965.
394. Wechsler, D.: *Wechsler Intelligence Scale for Children Manual.* New York Psychological Corp., 1949.
395. Wechsler, D.: *The Measurement and Appraisal of Adult Intelligence.* Baltimore, Williams & Wilkins, 1958.
396. Wechsler, D.: *The Wechsler Pre-School and Primary Scale of Intelligence.* New York, Psychological Corp., 1967.
397. Dunn, L. M.: *Expanded Peabody Picture Vocabulary Test.* Minneapolis, American Guidance Assoc., 1965.
398. Justak, J. F. and Jastak, S. R.: *The Wide Range Achievement Test.* Willmington, Guidance Assoc., 1965.
399. Myklebush, H.: *Development and Disorders of Written Language.* Vol. I: Picture Story Test. New York, Grune & Stratton, 1965.
400. Glaser, K. and Clemens, R. L.: School failure. *Pediatrics, 35:*128, 1963.
401. Leton, D. H.: Discriminant analysis of WISC profiles of learning disabled and culturally disadvantaged pupils. *Psychol School, 9:*303, 1972.
402. Rise, D. B.: Learning disabilities, an investigation in two patients parts, part I. *J Learn Dis, 3:*149, 1970.
403. Ruzel, R. P.: WISC subtest scores of disabled readers: A view with respect to Bannatyne's recategorization. *J Learn Dis, 7:*57, 1974.
404. Wepman, J.: *Auditory Discrimination Tests.* Chicago, University of Chicago Press, 1958.

405. Shields, D.: Brain response to stimuli in disorders of information processing. *J Learn Dis, 6:*501-505.

406. Regan, D.: *Evoked Potentials in Psychology, Sensory Physiology and Clinical Medicine.* New York, Wiley-Interscience, 1972.

407. Guyer, P. L. and Friedman, M. P.: Hemispheric processing and cognitive styles in learning disabled and normal children. *Child Dev, 46:*658, 1975.

408. Conners, C. K.: Cortical visual evoked response in children with learning disorders. *Psychophysiology, 7:*418, 1971.

409. Ayers, A. J.: *Sensory Integration and Learning Disorders.* Los Angeles, Western Psychological Service, 1972.

410. Yamada, I., Kimura, J., Young, S., and Paneus, M.: Somatosensory evoked potentials elicited by bilateral stimulation of the median nerve and its clinical application. *Neurology, 28:*218, 1978.

411. Smith, O. W. and Smith, P. C.: Developmental studies of spatial judgements by children and adults. *Percept Mot Skills, 22:*3, 1966.

412. Silberberg, N. E. and Silberberg, M. C.: Myths in remedial education. *J Learn Dis, 2:*209, 1969.

413. Hermann, K.: *Reading Disability.* Springfield, Thomas, 1959.

414. Thompson, L. J.: *Reading Disability – Developmental Dyslexia.* Springfield, Thomas, 1966.

415. Keeney, A. H. and Keeney, V. T.: *Diagnosis and Treatment of Reading Disorders.* St. Louis, Mosby, 1968.

416. Kinsbourne, M.: Models of learning disability: Their relevance to remediation. *Can Med Assoc J, 113:*1066, 1969.

417. Silver, L. B.: Acceptable and controversial approaches to treating the child with learning disabilities. *Pediatrics, 55:*406, 1975.

418. Bakker, D. J. and Satz, P.: *Specific Reading Disability: Advances in Theory and Method.* Rotterdam, Rotterdam University Press, 1976.

419. Kinsbourne, M. and Warrington, E. K.: Developmental factors in reading and writing backwardness. *Br J Psychol, 541:*145, 1963.

420. Sallustro, F. and Atwell, C. W.: Body rocking, head banging and head rolling in normal children. *J Pediatr, 93:*704, 1978.

421. Wolpe, J. and Lazarus, A.: *Behavior Therapy Techniques.* New York, Pergamon Press, 1966.

422. Baer, D. M., Wolf, M. M., and Risley, T. R.: Some current dimensions of applied behavior analysis. *J Appl Behav Anal, 1:*91, 1968.

423. Bandura, A.: *Principles of Behavior Modification.* New York, Holt, Rinehart & Winston, 1969.

424. Gardner, W. F.: *Behavior Modification: Applications for Mental Retardation.* Chicago, Aldine-Atherton, 1971.

425. Drabman, R. S. and Jarvie, G.: Counseling parents of children with behavior problems: The use of extinction and time out techniques. *Pediatrics, 59:*78, 1977.

426. Lesch, M. and Nyhan, W. L.: A familial disorder of uric acid metabolism and central nervous system function. *Am J Med, 36:* 561, 1964.

427. Feinstein, S. C. and Walpert, E. A.: Juvenile manic-depressive illness: Clinical and therapeutic considerations. *J Am Acad Child Psychiat,* *12*:123, 1973.

428. Efron, D. (Ed.): *Psychopharmacology, a Review of Progress 1957-1967.* Washington, D.C., Public Health Service Publication No. 1836, 1968.

429. World Health Organization Research in Psychopharmacology: *A Report of a W.H.O. Scientific Group.* W.H.O. Tech Rep Sec No. 371, 1967.

430. Omenn, G. S.: Neurochemistry and behavior in man. *West J Med,* *125*:434, 1976.

431. Maskowitz, M. A. and Wurtman, R. J.: Catecholamines and neurologic diseases. *N Engl J Med, 293*:274, 1975.

432. Von Brücke, F. T. and Hornykrewicz, O.: *The Pharmacology of Psychotherapeutic Drugs.* New York, Springer-Verlag, 1969.

433. Forrest, I. S., Carr, C. J. and Usdin (Eds.): *Advances in Biochemical Psychopharmacology.* New York, Raven, 1974, vol. IX.

434. Saurkes, T. L.: *Biochemistry of Mental Disease.* New York, Harper & Row, 1962.

435. Coppen, A.: The biochemistry of affective disorders. *Br J Psychiatr,* *113*:1237, 1967.

436. Himwich, H. E. (Ed.): *Biochemistry, Schizophrenia and Affective Illnesses.* Baltimore, Williams & Wilkins, 1970.

437. Snyder, S. H., Banerger, S. P. Yamamura, H. E. and Greenberg, D.: Drugs, neurotransmitters and schizophrenia. *Science, 184*:1243, 1974.

438. Weil-Malkerke, H. and Szara, S. I.: *The Biochemistry of Functional and Experimental Psychoses.* Springfield, Thomas, 1971.

439. Schildkraut, J. J.: *Neuropsychopharmacology and the Affective Disorders.* Boston, Little Brown, 1970.

440. Lynn, E. J., Satloff, A. and Tinley, D. C.: Mania and the use of lithium. A three year study. *Am J Psychiat, 127*:1176, 1971.

441. Le Dain, G. (Chairman): *Interim Report on the Commission of Inquiry into the Non-Medical Use of Drugs.* Ottawa, Queen's Printer for Canada, 1970.

442. Meyers, F. H. and Solomon, P.: Psychopharmacology. In Solomon, P. and Patch, V. D. (Eds.): *Handbook of Psychiatry,* 3rd ed. Los Altos, Lange Medical Publications, 1974, pp. 427-436.

443. Sharpless, S. K.: Hypnotics and sedatives. I Barbiturates and II Miscellaneous agents. In Goodman, L. S. and Gillmore, A. (Eds.): *The Pharmacological Basis of Therapeutics,* 4th ed. London, Macmillian, 1970, pp. 98-134.

444. Jarvik, M. E.: Drugs used in the treatment of psychiatric disorders. In Goodman, L. S. and Gillman, A. (Eds.): *The Pharmacologic Basis of Therapeutics,* 4th ed. London, Macmillian, 1970, pp. 151-203.

445. Sourkes, T. L.: Psychopharmacology and biochemical theories of mental disorders. In Siegel, G. J., Allers, R. W., Katzman, R. and Agranoff,

B. W. (Eds.): *Basic Neurochemistry*, 2nd ed. Boston, Little Brown, 1976, pp. 705-736.

446. Singer, I. and Rotenberg, D.: Mechanisms of lithium action. *N Engl J Med, 289:*254, 1973.

447. Schaw, M.: Lithium in psychiatric therapy and prophylaxis. *J Psychiatr Rev, 6:*67, 1968.

448. Schaw, M. and Baastrup, D.: Lithium as a prophylactic agent. *Arch Gen Psychiat, 16:*162, 1967.

449. Ampola, M. G.: Phenylketonuria and other disorders of amino acid metabolism. *Pediatr Clin North Am, 20:*507, 1973.

450. Scriver, C. R. and Rosenberg, L. E.: Aminoacid metabolism and its disorders. *Major Probl Clin Pediatr, 10:*1, 1973.

451. Frempter, G. W.: Aminoacidurias due to inherited disorders of metabolism Part I & II. *N Engl J Med, 289:*835 & 895, 1973.

452. Kolodny, E. H.: Lysosomal storage diseases. *N Engl J Med, 294:*1217, 1976.

453. Vinkin, P. J. and Brwyn, F. W. (Eds.): *Handbook of Clinical Neurology: Leucodystrophies and Poliodystrophies.* Amsterdam, North Holland Publishing Company, 1970, vol. X.

454. Vinkin, P. J. and Brwyn, F. W. (Eds.): *Handbook of Clinical Neurology: Phacomatoses.* Amsterdam, North Holland Publishing Company, 1972, vol. XIV.

INDEX